Dr. Malhotra's Series

Step by Step®

Hospital Designing and Planning

Dr. Malhotra's Series

Step by Step®

Hospital Designing and Planning

Second Edition

Authors

Sangeet Sharma
B Arch, FIIA, MSc (Sustainable Development) PhD (USA)
Practising Architect, Chandigarh

Purnima Sharma
B Arch, FIIA, MSc (Construction Management)
Practising Architect, Chandigarh

Series Editors

Narendra Malhotra MD FICOG

Jaideep Malhotra MD FICOG

www.narendramalhotra.net
e-mail: mnmhagra10@dataone.in

JAYPEE

JAYPEE BROTHERS MEDICAL PUBLISHERS
The Health Sciences Publisher
New Delhi | London

Jaypee Brothers Medical Publishers (P) Ltd

Headquarters
EMCA House, 23/23-B Ansari Road,
Daryaganj New Delhi 110 002, India
Landline: +91-11-23272143,
+91-11-23272703
+91-11-23282021, +91-11-23245672
e-mail: jaypee@jaypeebrothers.com

Corporate Office
4838/24, Ansari Road,
Daryaganj New Delhi 110 002, India
Phone: +91-11-43574357
Fax: +91-11-43574314
e-mail: jaypee@jaypeebrothers.com

Overseas Office
JP Medical Ltd.
83, Victoria Street, London
SW1H 0HW (UK)
Phone: +44-20 3170 8910
e-mail: info@jpmedpub.com

EU GPSR Authorised Representative
Logos Europe, 9 rue Nicolas Poussin
17000, La Rochelle, France
Phone: +33 (0) 6 67 93 73 78
e-mail: contact@logoseurope.eu

Website: www.jaypeebrothers.com
Website: www.jaypeedigital.com

Inquiries for bulk sales may be solicited at: jaypee@jaypeebrothers.com

Step by Step® Hospital Designing and Planning

First Edition: 2007
Second Edition: 2010
Reprint: **2026**
ISBN 978-81-8448-820-3

Printed in India

Foreword

The first edition of Step by Step Hospital Designing and Planning was a hundred percent sell-out. We have strived to provide the medical fraternity with ready guide to plan the hospitals and nursing homes. We have now, with our experienced authors, come out with the updated second edition. Our experienced authors have contributed more information to make this book more useful.

This unique book on Hospital Designing and Planning is being presented to you under Dr Malhotra's Series of books.

Most of us are professional doctors who are usually too busy to pay attention to subtle planning of our clinics, nursing homes and hospitals. We doctors usually are our own architects and we build as need arises.

Architects Sangeet Sharma, Purnima Sharma; a dynamic husband-wife team of Chandigarh, are well versed with the needs of doctors and have to their credit the designing of big/small hospitals and clinics across India.

In this book Sangeet and Purnima present to you a stepwise approach to designing and building a clinic or a hospital.

Happy reading

Narendra Malhotra
Jaideep Malhotra
(Series Editors)

Preface to the Second Edition

The book *Step by Step Hospital Designing and Planning* is presented to you, keeping in mind all the national and international standards required. Most of our ideas, plans and our guidelines confer to ISO standards.

We hope this new edition with more information and photographs will help you design your clinic and hospital to the best.

If you want to heal and treat, you have to have surroundings that are pleasant, clean and cheerful.

Sangeet Sharma
Purnima Sharma

Preface to the First Edition

If you want to heal and treat, you have to have surroundings that are pleasant, clean and cheerful.

We are presenting this stepwise book for you, keeping in mind all the national and international standards required. Most of our ideas, plans and our guidelines confer to ISO standards.

We hope this small booklet will help you design your clinic and hospital to the best.

Sangeet Sharma
Purnima Sharma

Acknowledgements

We are delighted that the first print of this book was a complete sell-out and in our effort to provide more information, we are upgrading and updating the information for your benefit.

We once again thankfully acknowledge the trust Dr Narendra Malhotra bestowed upon us for doing the book. We will always be grateful to his vision, guidance and help all through the process of preparing this manual in particular to him and in general to Malhotra Nursing and Maternity Home, Agra, India.

We are grateful to "Journal of Indian Institute of Architects", Vol. 67, Issue 09 and experienced authors like GD Kundres, Ar Sumit Kalra, Ar Dr BS Bhushan, Ms P Meena Kumari, KK Mitra, SP Jain, CVR Murty for guiding us through their articles and written words. It is our endeavor that through this manual we will benefit all doctors and planners who wish to build their nursing homes and hospitals.

We also thank Dr RM Malhotra, Dr Prabha Malhotra and Dr Jaideep Malhotra for their encouragement and guidance. We also thank Ar SD Sharma and Mrs Geeta Sharma for their teaching support and guidance. We are thankful to Richa Sarin and Richa Tondon for their efforts in formation of this manual. We also acknowledge the contribution of Harvinder Singh, Meenakshi and Satwinder Singh for their constant support in bringing out this book. We are obliged to National Building Code and Newferts architects data for tables and other reference materials. We are thankful to M/s Jaypee Brothers Medical Publishers (P) Ltd., New Delhi, for entrusting us with this task of reproducing this manual.

Contents

Chapter 1

Introduction

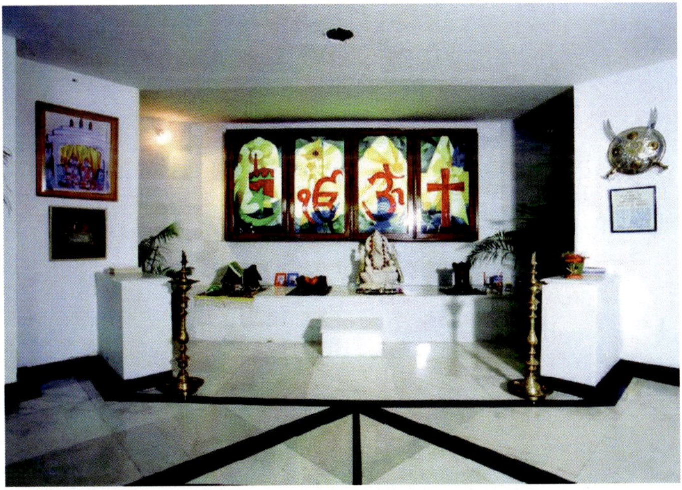

Encompassing motifs of all religions, this unique place of worship is at Silver Oak Hospital, Mohali, Punjab.

BASIC PRINCIPLES OF DESIGNS

Good design has no absolute formula, it is the successful employment of aesthetic principles and element:

- Scale and proportion
- Rhythm
- Balance
- Harmony
- Integrity and simplicity
- Good proportion
- Appropriateness of materials
- Structural design
- Color-use in hospital
- Lighting- artificial
- Natural
- Psychological effect.

RESPONSIBILITY OF DESIGNERS/ARCHITECT

1. In proper planning all principles are to be taken care of properly.
2. To coordinate all elements of design to create functionally and aesthetically.
3. Pleasing, healing environment to fulfill the total need of client or user.
4. To use every square feet so that cost is justified.
5. To visualize the last interior detail in the initial planning stage.
6. Knowledge of appropriate styles of architecture, furniture and styles.
7. Knowledge of materials to be used in construction, which are durable, maintenance free. All materials including floor wall, window upholstery should be well thought of.

Flow chart 1.1: Role of an architect

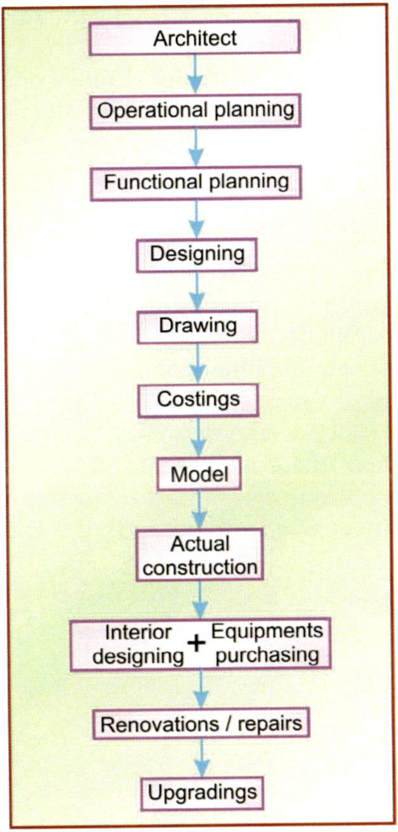

8. Lighting effects must be a mix of natural and artificial lights. Soothing colors have healing effects and spaces must be created considering these psychological aspects.

9. All services to be planned well in synchronization with all materials and design and to be comfortable to use.
10. To take responsibility till the completion of project, willing to see the flows in quality and understanding craftsmanship.
11. Able to incorporate artistry and expertise within clients purpose and objectives within bounds of good taste.
12. A designer should be a person with attributes including enthusiasm.
13. Imagination, curiosity perceptual skills, sociability, respects for time, commitments and organizational and record keeping skill.
14. In short designer/architect should be a person for whom there is liking, trust, faith and rapport. With whom one can design freely about all the views. A person who understands the client as well as the project.

Chapter 2

Hospitals: Facilities and Norms for Planning

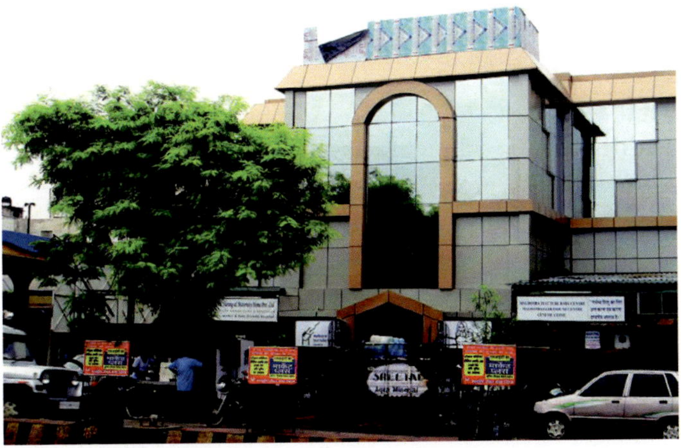

The prosperous Malhotra's nursing and Maternity Home at Agra.

NORMS AND STANDARDS IN HOSPITAL PLANNING

Table 2.1

Off - street parking spaces	*Institutional (Medical)*	
	Private	*Public*
Population less than 50000	20 beds	30
Population 50000 to 200000	15	25
Population between 200000 to 1000000	10	15
Population between 1000000 to 5000000	5	10
Population above 5000000	2	5

Corridors and Passageways

All means of exit including staircases, lifts, lobbies and corridors shall be adequately ventilated.

Internal Staircases

Minimum width for staircase shall be 2.0 m. The minimum width of tread without nosing shall be 250 mm for internal staircase of residential buildings. This shall be 300 m for institutional building. The treads shall be constructed and maintained in a manner to prevent slipping.

- Hydrotherapy = 4 sq. ft.
- Electrotherapy and exercise = 2.4 sq. ft.
- Occupational therapy and related services = 11.5 sq. ft.
  It includes :
  - OT = 4.2 sq. ft.
  - Sheltered workshop = 1.16 sq. ft.
  - Cerebral palsy treatment and training center. = 6.16 sq. ft.
- Outpatient department = 35.6 sq. ft.
  It includes :
  - Clinic = 6.83 sq. ft.
  - Reserve = 2.3 sq. ft.

- Dental and ENT = 8 sq. ft.
- EKC and BMR = 2.3 sq. ft.
- Medical social service = 5 sq. ft.
- Corridor and waiting room = 11.17 sq. ft.

- Pharmacy Medical
  - Social = 3.6 sq. ft.
- Service = 2.5 sq. ft.

Flow chart 2.1: Approach to building a hospital

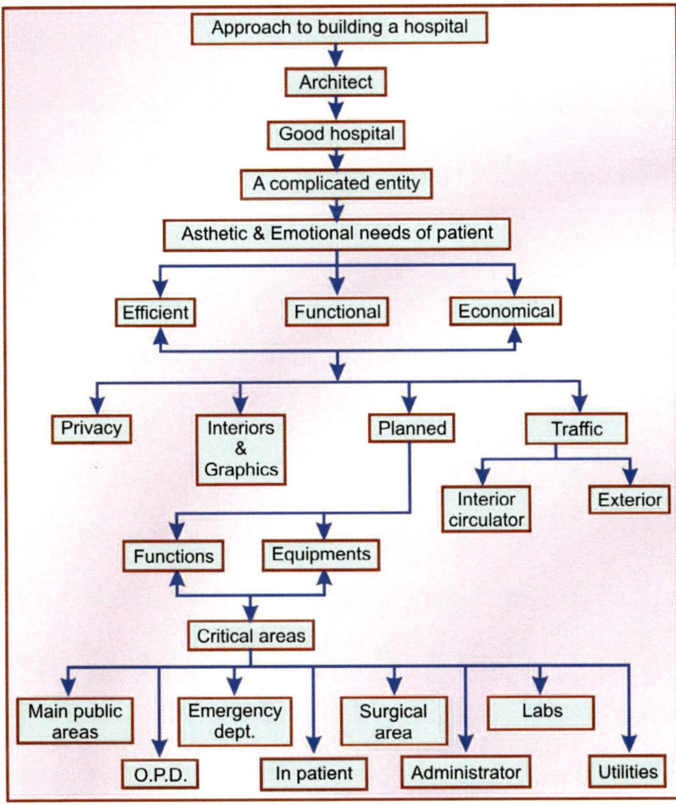

Table 2.2: Minimum requirements for Fire Fighting Installations: Institutional Buildings

S. No.	Type of Building Occupancy	Type of Installation								
		Fire Extin-guisher	*Hose Reel*	*Dry Riser*	*Wet Riser*	*Down – Comer*	*Yard Hydrant*	*Automatic Sprinkler System*	*Manually Operated Electric Fire Alarm Systems*	*Automatic Detection and Alarm System*
A.	**Hospitals, Sanatoria and Nursing Homes (C-1)**									
1.	Less than 15 m in height with plot area up to 1000 m^2									
i.	Up to ground plus one storey, with no beds	R	R	NR	NR	NR	NR	R	R	NR
ii.	Up to ground plus one storey with beds	R	R	NR	NR	R	NR	R	R	NR

Contd...

Contd...

		Type of Installation								
S. No.	*Type of Building Occupancy*	*Fire Extinguisher*	*Hose Reel*	*Dry Riser*	*Wet Riser*	*Down – Comer*	*Yard Hydrant*	*Automatic Sprinkler System*	*Manually Operated Electric Fire Alarm Systems*	*Automatic Detection and Alarm System*
iii.	Ground plus two or more storeys, with no beds	R	R	NR	NR	R	NR	R	R	NR
iv.	Ground plus two or more storeys, with beds	R	R	NR	R	NR	NR	R	R	R
2	Less than 15 m in height with plot area more than 1000 m^2	R	R	NR	R	NR	R	R	R	R
3.	15 m and above but not exceeding 24 m in height	R	R	NR	R	NR	R	R	R	R

Contd...

Contd...

		Type of Installation								
S. No.	*Type of Building Occupancy*	*Fire Extin-guisher*	*Hose Reel*	*Dry Riser*	*Wet Riser*	*Down – Comer*	*Yard Hydrant*	*Automatic Sprinkler System*	*Manually Operated Electric Fire Alarm Systems*	*Automatic Detection and Alarm System*
4.	Above 24 m and not exceeding 30 m in height	R	R	NR	R	NR	R	R	R	R
B.	**Custodial (C-2) and Penal and Plental (C-3)**									
1.	Less than 10 m in height									
i.	Upto 300 persons	R	R	NR	NR	NR	NR	R	R	NR
ii.	More than 300 persons	R	R	NR	NR	R	NR	R	R	NR
2.	10 m and above but not exceeding 15 m in height	R	R	NR	R	NR	R	R	R	R

Contd...

Contd...

S. No.	Type of Building Occupancy	*Type of Installation*								
		Fire Extinguisher	*Hose Reel*	*Dry Riser*	*Wet Riser*	*Down – Comer*	*Yard Hydrant*	*Automatic Sprinkler System*	*Manually Operated Electric Fire Alarm Systems*	*Automatic Detection and Alarm System*
3.	15 m and above but not exceeding 24 m in height	R	R	NR	R	NR	R	R	R	R
4.	24 m and above but not exceeding 30 m in height	R	R	NR	R	NR	R	R	R	R

R — Required
NR — Not required

Table 2.3: Public health services

	Type of Installation	*Water Supply (in l)*		*Pump Capacity (in l/min)*	
S. No.	*Type of Building Occupancy*	*Underground Static Water Storage Tank*	*Terrace Tank*	*Pump near Underground Static Water Storage Tank (Fire Pump) with Minimum Pressure of 3.5 kg/cm² at Terrace Level*	*At the Terrace Tank Level with Minimum pressure of 2.0 kg/cm²*
A.	**Hospitals, Sanatoria and Nursing Homes (C-1)**				
1.	Less than 15 m in height with plot area up to 1000 m²				
i.	Up to ground plus one storey, with no beds	NR	2500 (2500)	NR	NR
ii.	Up to ground plus one storey with beds	NR	5000 (5000)	NR	450(450)
iii.	Ground plus two or more storeys, with no beds	NR	5000(5000)	NR	450(450)
iv.	Ground plus two or more storeys, with beds	50000	5000 (5000)		NR
2.	Less than 15 m in height with plot area more than 1000 m²	100000	10000		NR
3.	15 m and above but				

Contd...

Contd...

Type of Installation		Water Supply (in l)		Pump Capacity (in l/min)	
S. No.	*Type of Building Occupancy*	*Underground Static Water Storage Tank*	*Terrace Tank*	*Pump near Underground Static Water Storage Tank (Fire Pump) with Minimum Pressure of 3.5 kg/cm^2 at Terrace Level*	*At the Terrace Tank Level with Minimum pressure of 2.0 kg/cm^2*
	not exceeding 24 m in height	100000	20000		NR
4.	Above 24 m and not exceeding 30 m in height	100000	20000		NR
B.	**Custodial (C-2) and Penal and Plental (C-3)**				
1.	Less than 10 m in height				
i.	Upto 300 persons	NR	10000 (5000)	NR	450 (900)
ii.	More than 300 persons	NR	15000 (5000)	NR	450 (900)
2.	10 m and above but not exceeding 15 m in height	50000	5000(5000)		NR
3.	15 m and above but not exceeding 24 m in height	75000	10000		NR
4.	24 m and above but not exceeding 30 m in height	100000	20000		NR

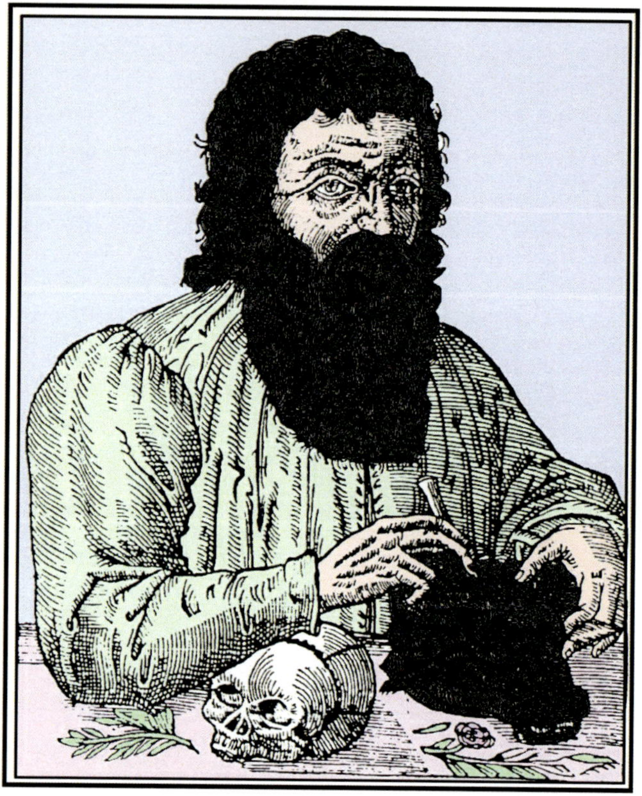

Fig. 2.1: Hippocrates (C 460-377 BC). Greek physician and the originator of the clinical study of medicine (The Beltman Archive)

REQUIREMENTS OF INSTITUTIONAL BUILDINGS

1. In buildings or sections occupied by bed-ridden patients where the floor area is over 280 m^2, facilities shall be provided to move patients in hospital beds to the other side of a smoke barrier from any part of such

building or section not directly served by approved horizontal exits or exits from the first floor (floor 2) of a building to the outside.

2. Not less than two exits of one or more of the following types shall be provided for every floor including basement, of every building or section:
   a. Doors leading directly outside the buildings;
   b. Stairways;
   c. Ramps;
   d. Horizontal exits; and
   e. Fire tower
3. All required exits that serve as egress from hospital or infirmary sections shall be not less than 2 m in clear width including patient bedroom doors to permit transportation of patients on beds, litters or mattresses. The minimum width of corridors serving patients bedrooms in buildings shall be 2400 mm.
4. Elevators constitute a desirable supplementary facility, but are not counted as required exits. Patient lifts shall also be provided with enough room for transporting a stretcher trolley.
5. Any area exceeding 500 m^2 shall be divided into compartments by fire resistant walls.
6. Doors in fire resistant walls shall be so installed that these may normally be kept in open position, but will close automatically. Corridor door openings in smoke barriers shall be not less than 2000 mm in width. Provision shall also be made for double swing single/ double leaf type door.
7. Exists and other features for penal and mental institutions, and custodial institutions shall be the same as specified for hospitals, in so far as applicable. Reliable means shall be provided to permit the prompt release

Flow chart 2.2: What makes a good hospital?

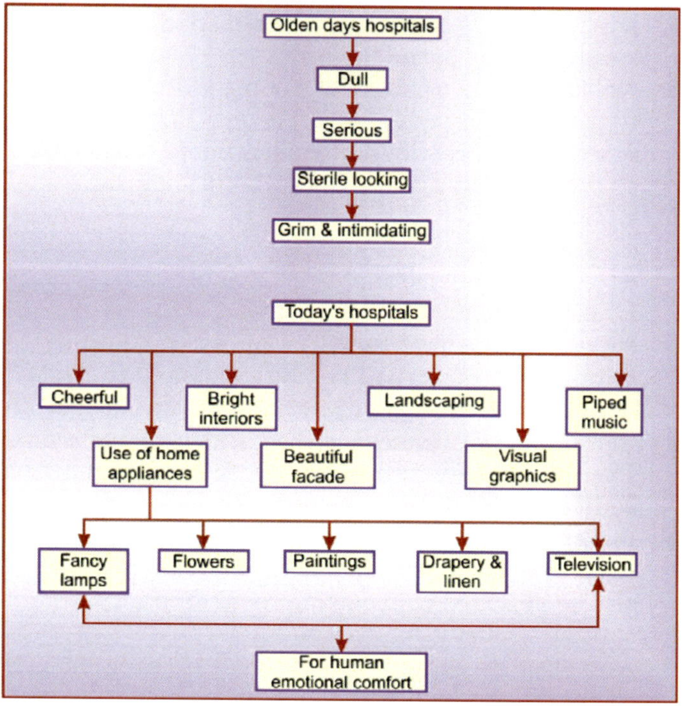

of inmates from any locked section in case of fire or other emergency.

8. Wherever any inmates are confined in any locked rooms or spaces, adequate guards or other personnel shall be continuously on duty or immediately available to provide for release of inmates or for such other action as may be indicated in case of fire or other emergency.
9. No building constructed in whole or in part of combustible materials shall be used to confine inmates in cells or sleeping quarters, unless automatic sprinkler protection is provided.

Additional Precautions

Bare minimum quantities of flammable material such as chloroform, ethyl alcohol, spirit, etc. shall be allowed to be stored and handled. The handling of such liquids shall not be permitted by un-authorized persons. Bulk storage of these items, will be governed by relevant rules and safe practices.

Exceptions and Deviations

It is recognized that in institutions or part of buildings housing various types of psychiatric patients or used as penal and mental institutions, it is necessary to maintain locked doors and barred windows; and to such extent the necessary provision in other sections of the code requiring the keeping of exits unlocked may be waived. It is also recognized that certain type of psychiatric patients are not capable of seeking safety without adequate guidance. In buildings where this situation prevails, reliable means for the rapid release of occupants shall be provided, such as remote control of locks, or by keying all locks to keys commonly used by attendants.

Flow chart 2.3: Good hospital

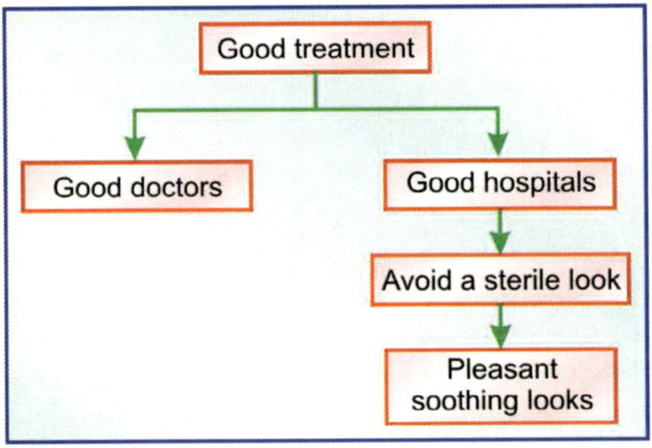

Table 2.4: Recommended values of illuminance

Type of Interior or Activity	*Range of Service Illuminance in Lux Hospitals*	*Quality Class of Direct Glare Limitation*	*Remarks*
Anesthetic rooms			
Ward corridors	150-200-300	—	
Day screened from bays	150-200-300	—	
Day, open to natural light	150-200-300 (Total)	—	
Treatment	750-1000-1500	—	
Examination			
General	200-300-500	—	
Local inspection	750-1000-1500	—	
Intensive therapy			
Bad head	30-50		
Circulation between bed ends	50-100-150	—	
Observation	200-300-500	—	
Local observation	750-1000-1500	—	
Staff base (day)	200-300-500	—	
Staff base (night)	30	—	
Nurse's station			
Night medical trolleys	50-100-150		
Operation theaters			
General	30-500-750	—	
Local	10000 to 50000	—	
Special operating lights are used Pathology Department			
General	200-300-500	—	
Examination	300-500-750	—	
Pharmacies	20-300-500	—	
Reception/enquiry	200-300-500	—	
Recovery rooms	200-300-500	—	
Ward circulation			
Ward-bed head			

Contd...

Contd...

Type of Interior or Activity	*Range of Service Illuminance in Lux Hospitals*	*Quality Class of Direct Glare Limitation*	*Remarks*
Pediatric	1		
Psychiatric	1-5		
X-ray areas			
General	150-200-300		
Diagnostic	150-200-300		
Operative	200-300-500		
Process dark room	50		
Surgeries			
General	200-300-500	—	
Waiting rooms	100-150-200	—	
Dental surgeries			
Consulting rooms			
General	200-300-500	—	
Ophthalmic wall and near-vision charts	300-500-750	—	
Medical First Aid center			
Consulting rooms, Treatment rooms	300-500-750	1	
Rest rooms	100-150-200	1	
Medical stores	100-150-200	2	

RECOMMENDED VALUE FOR AIR CHANGES

The standards of general ventilation are recommended/ based on maintenance of required oxygen, carbon dioxide and other air quality levels and for the control of body odours when no products of combustion or other contaminants are present in the air; the values of air changes should be shown in Table 2.5.

Table 2.5: Outdoor air requirements for ventilation of air conditioned areas and commercial facilities

Application	*Estimated maximum occupancy*	*Outdoor air requirement*		*Remarks*
		l/s/person	*(l/s)/m²*	
Hospital, nurses and convalescent homes				
Patient rooms	10	13		Special requirements or codes provisions and pressure relationships may determine minimum ventilation rates and filter efficiency.
Medical procedure	20	8		
Operating rooms	20	15		
Procedure recovery and ICU		20	8	Generating contaminants may require higher rates.
			2.50	Air shall not be re-circulated into other spaces.
Autopsy				
Physical therapy	20	8		
Correctional cells	20	10		
Dinning halls	100	8		
Guard stations	40	8		

Hospitals/Operating Theaters

In many cases proper air conditioning can be a factor in the therapy of the patient and in some instances part of the major treatment. For special application areas of

Flow chart 2.4: Circulation

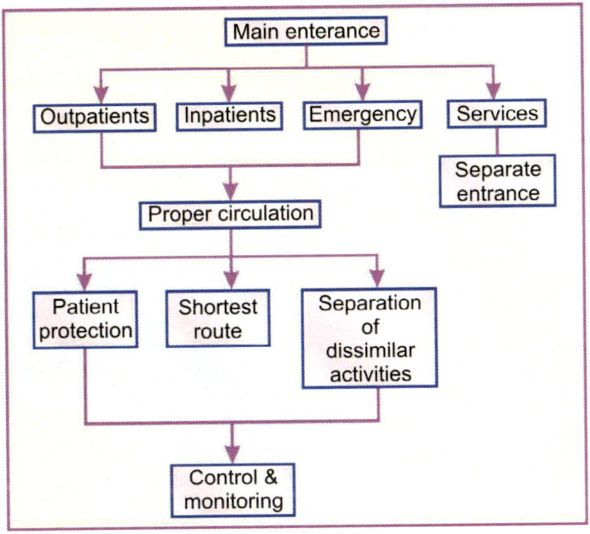

hospitals such as operation theaters, reference may be made to specialist literature.

The main difference in application compared with other applications are:

a. Restriction of air movement between various departments and control of air movement within certain departments, to reduce the risk of air-borne cross infection;
b. Specific need for the ventilation and filtration equipment to dilute and/or remove particulate or gaseous contamination and air-borne micro-organisms;
c. Close tolerances in temperatures and humidities may be required for various areas; and
d. The design should allow for accurate control of environmental conditions.

Acceptable Indoor Noise Level dB (A) for Hospitals is 35-40

Hospital Bed Lifts: Hospital bed lifts should be situated conveniently near the ward and operating theater entrances. There shall be sufficient space near the landing door for easy movement of stretcher.

It is convenient to place the passenger lifts in a hospital, near the staircases.

Water Requirement for Hospitals

Type of Building	*Consumption Per day, liters*
Hospitals (including Laundry):	
a. Number of beds not exceeding 100	340 per head
b. Number of beds exceeding 100	450 per head

Table 2.6: Hospitals with indoor patient wards

S. No.	*Fixtures*	*Patient toilets*		*Staff toilets*	
		Male	*Female*	*Male*	*Female*
i.	Toilet suite comprising one wc and one washbasin and shower stall	Private room with up to 4 patients		For individual doctor's/officer's rooms	
	For General Wards, Hospital Staff and Visitors				
ii.	Water-closets	1 per 8 beds or part thereof	1 per 8 beds of part thereof.	1 for up to 152 for 16-35	1 for up to 122 for 13-25
iii.	Ablution tap	One in each water-closet	One in each water-closet	One in each water-closet	One in each water-closet.
		1 water tap with draining arrangements shall be provided for every 50 persons or part thereof in the vicinity of water-closets and urinals.			
iv.	Urinals	1 per 30 beds	—	Nil up to 6 1 for 7 to 20 2 for 21-45	—
v.	Washbasins	2 for every 30 beds or part thereof. Add 1 per additional 30 beds or part thereof		1 for up to 15 2 for 16-35	1 for up to 12 2 for 13-25
vi.	Drinking water fountain	1 per ward		1 per 100 persons or part thereof	
vii.	Cleaner's sink	1 per ward		—	
viii.	Bed pan sink	1 per ward		—	
ix.	Kitchen sink	1 per ward		—	

Table 2.7: Hospitals outdoor patient department

S. No.	Fixtures	Patient toilets		Staff toilets	
		Male	*Female*	*Male*	*Female*
i.	Toilet suite comprising one wc and one washbasin (with optional shower stall if building used for 24 h)	For up to 4 patients		For individual doctor's/officer's rooms	
ii.	Water closets	1 per 100 persons or part thereof	2 per 100 persons or part thereof	1 for up to 15 2 for 16-35	1 for up to 12 2 for 13-25
iii.	Ablution tap	One in each water-closet	One in each water-closet	One in each water-closet	One in each water-closet
		1 water tap with draining arrangements shall be provided for every 50 persons or part thereof in the vicinity of water-closets and urinals			
iv.	1 Urinals	1 per 50 persons or part thereof	—	Nil up to 6 1 for 7 to 20 2 for 21-45	—
v.	Washbasins	1 per 100 persons or part thereof	2 per 100 persons or part thereof	1 for up to 15 2 for 16-35	1 for up to 12 2 for 13-25
vi.	Drinking water fountain	1 per 500 persons or part thereof		1 per 100 persons or part thereof	

Table 2.8: Administrative Buildings

S. No.	Fixtures	Staff toilets	
		Male	*Female*
i.	Toilet suite comprising one wc and one washbasin (with optional shower stall if building used for 24 h)	For individual doctor's/officer's rooms	
ii.	Water - closets	1 per 25 persons or part thereof	1 per 15 persons or part thereof
iii.	Ablution tap	One in each water-closet	One in each water-closet
		1 water tap with draining arrangements shall be provided for every 50 persons or part thereof in the vicinity of water-closets and urinals	
iv.	Urinals	Nil up to 6 1 for 7 to 20 2 for 21 – 45	—
v.	Washbasins	1 per 25 persons or part thereof	1 per 25 persons or part thereof
vi.	Drinking water fountain	1 per 100 persons or part thereof	
vii.	Cleaner's sink	1 per floor, *Min*	
viii.	Kitchen sink	1 per floor, *Min*	

Table 2.9: Hospitals staff quarters and nurses homes

S. No.	Fixtures	*Staff quarters*		*Nurses homes*	
		Male	*Female*	*Male*	*Female*
i.	Water-closets	1 per 4 persons or part thereof	1 per 4 persons or part thereof	1 per 4 persons or part thereof 2 for 16-35	1 per 4 persons or part thereof 2 for 13-25
ii.	Ablution tap	One in each water-closet	One in each water-closet	One in each water-closet	One in each water-closet
		1 water tap with draining arrangements shall be provided for every 50 persons or part thereof in the vicinity of water-closets and urinals			
iii.	Washbasins	1 per 8 persons or part thereof		1 per 8 persons or part thereof	
iv.	Bath (Showers)	1 per 4 persons or part thereof		1 per 4 to 6 persons or part thereof	
v.	Drinking water fountain	1 per 100 persons or part thereof, minimum 1 per floor		1 per 100 persons or part thereof, minimum1 per floor	
vi.	Cleaner's sink	1 per floor		1 per floor	

NOTES

1. Some WC's may be European style if desired.
2. For independent housing units fixtures shall be provided as for residences.

Table 2.10: List of rooms and space requirements

No.	Description	Area Sft.	Remarks
1.	Laboratory Superintendent's office-cum-research room with toilet attached	200	Only in hospitals of 200 beds and more
2.	General laboratory	300 to 400	——
3.	Washing and sterilizing	120 to 150	In hospitals of 100 beds and more
4.	EKG, BMR, specimen room	200 to 240	- do -
5.	Bacteriology and serology	200 to 240	In hospitals of 200 beds and more
6.	Storage	80 to 120	In hospitals of 100 beds and more.
7.	Reception area	120 to 150	-do-

Flow chart 2.5: Critical areas of hospital

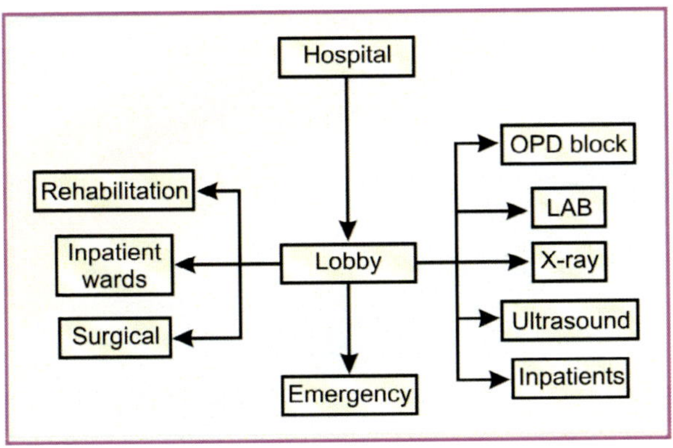

Table 2.11: Optimum sizes of rooms

No.	*Name of facility*	*Size in sft.*
	Surgical	
1.	Consultation room (Single Cubicle)	160
2.	Dressing room (with two tables)	180
3.	Waiting space (Minimum)	150
4.	Subsidiary waiting space	8 per patient
	Medical	
5.	Examination room	150
6.	Waiting space	8 per patient
	E.N.T.	
7.	Consultation room	150 to 180
8.	Treatment room	100 to 120
9.	Waiting space	8 per patient
	Eye Clinic	
10.	*Consultation room	150 to 180
11.	*Refraction room	200 to 240
12.	*Perimeter room	120
13.	*Tonography room	120
14.	*Slit-lamp room	120
15.	Orthoptics	150 each room
	****Planning**	
16.	Diagnostic room	180
17.	Treatment room	2 cubicles each of 120
	V.D. and Skin Clinics	
18.	Consultation and examination room	150 to 180 for each clinic
19.	Treatment room	2 cubicles each of 120
	Orthopedic Clinic	
20.	Consultation room	180
21	Plaster preparation room	120
22.	Fracture and treatment room	180
23.	Recovery room	120
24.	Waiting space	10 per patient

Contd...

Contd...

No.	Name of facility	Size in sft.
	Dental Clinic	
25.	Consultation examination and X-ray room	180
26.	Office room	120
27.	Recovery room	120 to 150
	Pediatric Clinic	
28.	Consultation and examination room	150
29.	Dressing, treatment and dispensary 120 for smaller hospitals	260 for bigger hospitals of 500 beds or above
	Psychiatry	
30.	Consultation room	120 to 150
31.	Room for social worker and record storage	150
32.	Examination room	
33.	Treatment room	Min. 160 for one bed.
	Infectious Diseases Clinic	
34.	Examination and treatment room	300
	Accident and Emergency Deptt.	
35.	Reception hall	150 to 250
36.	Reception counter with toilet facilities	150
37.	Examination room	Two cubicles each of 80
38.	X-Ray examination	80
39.	Laboratory	120
40.	Treatment room	150 to 300
41.	Operating room	Minor – 324 Major –600
42.	Ward attached to minor operation theaters	@ 70 sft. Per bed including toilet facilities
	Emergency Ward	@ 80 per bed
43.	Ambulance vehicle garage	@ 200 per vehicle
44.	Doctor's duty-cum-retiring room	160
46.	Stores	200
47.	Retiring room for drivers	160

Contd...

Contd...

No.	Name of facility	Size in sft.
	Dispensary (Pharmacy)	
48.	Waiting hall	@ 8 sft. Per head of 5% of the total clinical visits.
49.	Dispensing room	120-320
50.	Medicine stores	100 to 200
	Injection clinic	
51.	Injection room	120 to 160
	Blood Bank	
52.	Reception room	120 to 160
53.	Bleeding room	120 to 160
54.	Laboratory	120 to 240
55.	Recovery room	120 to 150
56.	Storage	36
57.	Washing and sterilizing	80 to 100
58.	Office room	120
	laboratories	
59.	Laboratory superintendent's.	200
60.	General laboratory	300 to 400
61.	Washing and sterilizing	120 to 150
62.	EKG, BMR, specimen room	200 to 240
63.	Bacteriology and serology	200 to 240
64.	Storage	80 to 120
65.	Reception area	120 to 150
	General	
66.	Entrance hall	400 to 2,000 sft. Or @ 1 sft. For one patient
67.	Tea Bar	120
	Administration	
68.	Medical Superintendent's room with 200 beds or more	180 only in Hospitals
69.	Janitor's room	40
	Storages	
70.	Drug Stores	300 or more

* These specifications are meant for an independent Eye Hospital.
** These specifications are for a General Hospital having Eye Clinic.

Lighting

Table 2.12

Sr. No.	*Location*	*Average lumens per sft. recommended at working level*
1.	General ward lighting	3*
2.	Minimum in center of ward	10
3.	Bed-head lighting, Nurse's station, day space	15
4.	Treatment rooms	20
5.	Sister's and Doctor's room	15
6.	Ward kitchen	10
7.	Sluice room	7
8.	Bath room and lavatories	5
9.	Cleaner's rooms, corridors and stair cases	5
10.	Waiting rooms	7

Number and Size of Theaters

Table 2.13

S.No.	*Total No. of beds*	*Number of theater units*			
		Main Operating Deptt.		*O.P.D.*	
		Major	*Minor*	*Major*	*Minor*
1.	25	1	—	—	1
2.	50	1	—	—	1
3.	75	1	1	—	1
4.	100	1	1	—	1
5.	300	3	1	—	1
6.	500	5	2	1	1
7.	750	8	2	1	1
8.	1000	10	2	1	1

The Space Requirement of the Central Sterilization and Supply Department

Table 2.14

Facility	*Bed Strength*					
	50	100	200	500	750	1000
General						
a. Administration Office	—	—	120	120	120	120
b. Store room (new and unsterile)	120	240	160	240	240	240
Sterilization Unit						
a. Wash up area with a counter to receive used goods	120	120	180	180	240	240
b. Check up and assembly	180	180	240	240	320	320
c. Autoclave room	80	80	120	120	160	160
d. Storage and issue section	120	120	180	180	240	240
Total	**620**	**740**	**1000**	**1080**	**1320**	**1320**
Solution Preparation Unit						
a. Glass washing etc.	120	120	120	180	180	180
b. Solution preparation	120	120	120	180	180	180
c. Solution storage and Issue	120	120	120	180	180	180
Total	**360**	**360**	**360**	**540**	**540**	**540**
Over all total of floor area	**980**	**1100**	**1360**	**1620**	**1860**	**1860**

The size of the cubicles and wards may be as follows:-

Table 2.15

S.No.	*Cubicle/Ward*	*Size Sft.*	*Area per bed sft.*
i.	Single-bedded room	120	120
ii.	Two-bedded room	180	90
iii.	Three bedded cubicle	240	80
iv.	Four-bedded cubicle	320	80
v.	Six-bedded cubicle	480	80
vi.	Eight bedded cubicle	640	80
vii.	Twelve-bedded ward	960	80
viii.	Sixteen-bedded ward	1280	80

Nursery

Healthy babies are kept with the mothers. However, certain proportion of the children are born premature and an equal proportion of children fall sick, who require intensive care. The proportion of these children may be ascertained in the following manner for a ward of 20 maternity beds.

Steps

1. Average stay of mothers = 7 days
2. Total number of beds in the ward = 20
3. Total expected live births $\frac{20 \times 365}{7}$ = 1040
4. Premature infants 10% of 1040 = 104
5. Average stay of premature children = 30 days
6. Full term infants: $\frac{(1040 - 104)}{365} = \frac{936 \times 7}{365}$ = 18
7. Premature bassinets 104/12 = 9
8. Suspect bassinets = 10% of 18 = 2

Area Schedule for Hospitals of Different Bed Strength

Table 2.16

S. No.	*Stores*	*Description*		*No. of Beds*	
		1000	750	500	250
1.	Provision	400	320	240	160
2.	Vegetables store	80	60	40	40
3.	Meat store	40	40	40	40
4.	Milk store	60	60	40	40
5.	Day-to-day store	60	60	40	40
6.	Equipment store	240	160	120	120
7.	Fuel store	240	180	150	150
8.	Suppliers' store	120	120	120	120
9.	Janitor's store	60	60	60	60
	Total	1300	1060	850	770

Water Requirements According to I.S.I. Standards

Table 2.17

Type of Buildings	*Consumption per head per day (liters)*
i. Hospitals (including laundry) per bed	
a. Number of beds not exceeding 100	340
b. Number of beds exceeding 100	455
ii. Nurses homes and medical quarters	135
iii. Hostels (per bed)	180
iv. Residences Office	45
v. Residences	135

Sanitation for In-patient Wards

Table 2.18

Fitments	*For men and women*
Water-closets	1 for every 8 beds or part thereof
Ablution taps	1 in each water-closet plus one water tap with draining arrangements in the vicinity and water-closets and urinals for every 50 beds or part thereof.
Washbasins	2 upto 30 beds; and 1 for every additional 30 beds or part thereof.
Baths	1 bath with shower for every 8 beds or part thereof.
Bed pan washing sinks	1 for each ward
Cleaner's sinks	1 for each ward
Kitchen sinks and dish washers	1 for each ward

Sanitation for Out-patient Department

Table 2.19

Fitments	*For men*	*For women*
Water closets	1 for every 100 persons or part thereof	2 for every 100 persons
Ablution taps	1 in each water closet. 1 water tap with draining arrangements shall be provided for every 50 persons or part thereof in the vicinity of water closets and urinals.	1 in each water closet
Urinals	1 for every 50 persons or part thereof.	
Washbasins	4 for every 100 persons or part thereof.	1 for every 100 persons or part thereof.

Land

The land requirement of hospitals of 25 to 100 beds is indicated below. It is based on the consideration that one-third of the area will be covered by the hospital buildings, one-third by residential quarters and the remaining be left open.

Beds	Area (Acres)
25	5 - 7
50	8 - 10
75	10 - 15
100	15 - 20

Residential Accommodation

Table 2.20

Sr. No.	Type	Designation	Scale of accommodation		Remarks
			Floor Area Sft.	Plinth Area Sft.	
1.	V	Superintendent of the Hospital (Large Hospitals)	1650	2000	Single storey detached.
				2100	Double storey detached.
				450	Servant quarters
				225	Garages
2.	IV	Resident Medical Officer and Senior Assistant Medical Officer	1450	1750	Single storey semi-detached.
				1850	Double storey semi-detached.
				225	Garages
3.	III	Junior Medical Officers	1000	1200	Single storey semi-detached.

Contd...

Contd...

Sr. No.	Type	Designation	Scale of accommodation		Remarks
			Floor Area Sft.	Plinth Area Sft.	
				1280	Double storey semi-detached
4.	II	Technicians and Clerks	520	625	Single storey semi-detached.
				700	Double storey semi-detached.
5.	I	Inferior Servants (Class IV staff)	240	345	Single storey semi detached.
				370	Double storey semi-detached.

Means of Escape, Fire Protection, Hazardous Materials

Up to 2 hours needed evacuate 6—patients from 2-storey, 4 hours from 11-storey building: exhausting exercise for rescuers. All health buildings which contain high proportion of bedfast, disabled and confused patients should be low rise, preferably with patients restricted to ground and first floors.

Fire Compartments

Horizontal distance to alternative routes must not exceed 64 m.

Horizontal distance in single direction to exit must not exceed 15 m.

Travel distance within escape stairway must not exceed 45 m along going.

Fire Sub-compartments (Patient areas)

Floor area must not exceed 750 m^2.

Horizontal distance to alternative routes must not exceed 32 m.

Horizontal distance to single directional exit must not exceed 15 m.

Maximum occupancy 40 patients.

WARD DESIGN: ACUTE

Walking distance: Keep walking distances short as possible for nurses and ambulant patient. Maximum distance from bed to wc 12 m and from nurse working room to furthest bed approximate 20 m.

Observation: Continuous observation of patient by staff essential part of nursing care: during day achieved mainly in course of walking from one duty to another, at night from nurses station. Good design aim: 50 percent of beds to be visible from nurses station. Patients gain confidence from seeing staff at work, dead-leg wards not popular for this reason; if staff have no duty perform less likely visit ward.

Control: Patients, particularly children, adolescents and confused, need to be controlled; babies must not be too isolated from rest of ward. Mixed-sex wards have own control problems. Staff need to control visitors and check that they do not overtire patients.

Noise: Problem in large open areas; telephones and other mechanical equipment can be noisier than acceptable. Design for 40-45 dB by day and 35-40 dB at night in multi-B wards; 1-B wards should be 35-40 dB at all times. Courtyard designs can create problems of noise from adjacent windows.

Daylight and glare: Windows should not cause glare in bedfast patients' eyes; beds should be parallel to windows unless brise-soleil, external or between-glass blinds or similar devices fitted. Windows design important: confused patients may try get out; all opening lights should have device restricting accessible opening to 100.

Table 2.21

1-B rm	10.0 m^2	Excluding wc and shower depending on amount of day space provided in wards or as separate day space: separate 10.0 m^2 extra space for lockers etc.
Multi-B bay (per B)	9.3–10.0 m^2	
Dayr (per B)	0.75 m^2	
Lockers etc (per B)	0.5–1.0 m^2	
Nurse station	4.0-10.0 m^2	Based on storage only
Clean utility	10.2–18.0 m^2	
Dirty utility and sluice	14.0–16.0 m^2	
Treatment room	14.0–16.0 m^2	Depending on storage provided
Assisted bathroom	10.25-12.0 m^2	
Sister room	7.0–9.0 m^2	
Doctors room	7.0–9.0 m^2	
bathroom	7.0 m^2	For ambulant patients
Washing and shower compartment	2.75 m^2	
Wc with hand rinse basin	2.0–3.0 m^2	Min for ambulant PMax for wheelchair P
pantry	4.0–6.0 m^2	Beverage & snack point only
Wards	20.0 m^2	For ward service
Flower bay	2.0–2.5 m^2	
cleaner	5.0–8.0 m^2	
Storage (inc large equipment)	12.0–20.0 m^2	May be shared with another ward
Interview room and overnight stay	10.0 - 12.0 m^2	
Circulation area	25-40%	Depends on ward layout

ACUTE WARD: SUGGESTED AREAS LONG STAY WARDS

Now few completely bedfast patients needing bedpans and bed baths during day: majority will be taken to wc and bathroom even if incapable of attending to themselves. Because incontinence prevalent extra wc required aid training (maximum distance from furthest bed or corner of day area: 10 m). Where space limited omit treatment room and replace by cleansing room with bathroom or wc each with thermostatically controlled shower handset. WC, sluice and cleansing room must have efficient mechanical extract ventilation. Small utility room with washing machine and clothes drier needed for patients' clothes.

Provide extra storage space for wheelchairs, walking aids and sanichairs, and for greater supply of linen, incontinence pads and, where used, disposable bedpans and urinals. Cupboards also required for patients' suitcases and clothes not in current use, and for occupational therapy equipment.

All floor finishes should be soft, non-slip and washable plastic flooring with welded joints suitable for wc, bathroom and all nurse working areas. Carpets may be used in wards and daycare where number of incontinent patients are limited.

Mentally handicapped often also physically handicapped may also be noisy, aggressive, overactive and self destructive. Particularly important that furnishing be soft, spongeable and durable for these patients and that ceilings have should absorbent finish.

Long stay patients highly dependent on staff in cases of emergency: vital fire escape routes be easily identified, fire stop doors have automatic door closers.

Elevator level coding system using colors and numbers; helpful to patient with sensory defects; raised numerals aid near-sighted or blind.

ENTRANCE FOR NON-AMBULANT CASUALTIES AND OUTPATIENTS

Design area between 2 sets of doors to take trolley pushed by staff member, without obstruction from door swings, etc. (2700 clear). Integrate 3 dirt control zones into design. Provide canopy or recess doorway to shelter doors. If ambulance required to back up to door allow 3200 to underside of canopy.

ACCIDENT AND EMERGENCY

Generous storage required for stretchers, blankets and trolleys. For benefit of patients, relatives and escorts, who may be in severe state of shock, all waiting spaces as well as clinical areas should be heated to min 21°C.

CASUALTY DEPARTMENT

Patients come without appointment and may have to wait some time before being examined and treated; provide generous waiting space, with beverage point and at least 4 wc, 2 suitable for wheelchair users.

RADIOLOGY DEPARTMENTS

Separation of inpatient, typically on trolley, stretcher or wheelchair, from outpatient in street clothes and often bloody, should be maintained as long as possible, certainly through entrance, reception and waiting: if department large enough also through radiographic procedure and exit.

Flow chart 2.6: Placement of physiotherapy and occupational therapy area

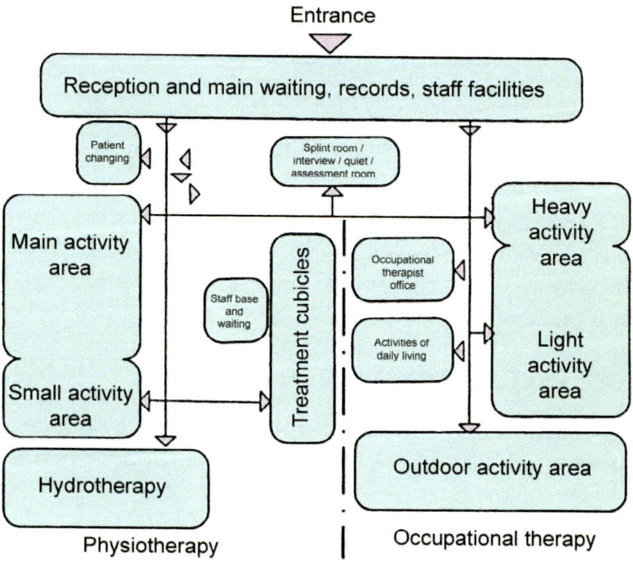

Arrange X-ray procedure room so that patient's travel path does not cross that of radiology technician until they meet in procedure room. Easy trolley/stretcher access to X-ray table essential.

OPERATING THEATERS

Surgical and delivery suites increasingly considered centers to which patients brought for procedures too complex for handling in physician's off or treatment area. Unlike traditional suite with different room for different services (eg. ENT, orthopedic) suites now collection of multi-purpose room. In large institutions more than 1 suite likely to be provided, based on usage: short (1-3 hr) procedures, such as ambulatory, frequently separated from general, average length (2-4 hr) and very long (6-8 hr) procedures. Delivery suites, formerly completely separated from surgical, today commonly alongside or integrated.

Space Needs

Space suites need per inpatient bed varies greatly, depending on whether ambulatory surgery offered, whether hospital has teaching program and other such factors: generally 28-46 m^2 for each operating theater.

Waiting

Provide general waiting area. Small forward waiting areas required for each group of consult room. Assuming appointment system, allow 7.0 m^2 waiting area for each suite. Seating should be comfortable and informal.

AREA ANALYSIS FOR HOSPITALS WITH BEDS 100 AND ABOVE

- Administration = 31.43 sq. ft.
- Surgical layout (central sterile, fracture room, surgery, dressing room, storage and office, corridor, staircase).
- For 1 bed,
  - Central sterile = 5.1 sq. ft.
  - Cystoscopy = 2.5 sq. ft.
  - Fracture room = 4.2 sq. ft.
  - Surgery = 13.52. sq. ft.
  - Dressing room + Storage = 5.6 sq. ft.
  - Office corridor + Stairs = 9.08 sq. ft.

- Special services = 18.45 sq. ft.
- For 1 bed.
  - Dental = 6.00 sq. ft.
  - ENT = 6.00 sq. ft.
  - EK4, BMR = 3.45 sq. ft.
  - Orthopedic and Oxygen therapy equipment = 3.00 sq. ft.
- Pathology, and clinical lab = 12.5 sq. ft.
- This includes
  - Lab = 8.5. sq. ft.
  - Morgue = 4 sq. ft.
- Radiology = 18 sq. ft.
- Physical therapy and rehabilitation = 6.4sq. ft.

Chapter 3

Services–The Backbone of Hospitals

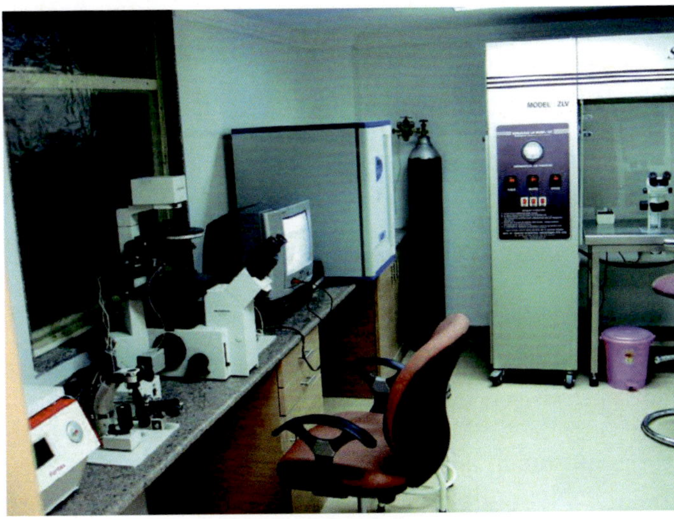

A typical view of the laboratory
(A.R.T. Lab)

The defects in hospital construction are the major concern for the hospital promoters. A lack of systematic planned approach to hospital functional and service planning is generally known to be a major reason for the defect. The functional analysis refers to the identification of the functions, the functional unit is going to perform, the location of functional unit, their design consideration; whereas the service parameters endeavours to conformance of implied requirements, thus attaining the objective of defect-free hospital. In essence, both functional analysis and framing of service requirements are the inherent characteristics of hospital design approach to eliminate the defects, which occur due to uncertainties. Their integration in the pre-construction stage shall further prevent the defects, which may occur because of the complexities in construction processes, the overlap of services, etc. This paper presents the functional approach of framing of functional and service requirements and integrating the two in pre-construction stage to achieve the defect-free hospital design.

INTRODUCTION

The technological advances made in the recent past have introduced many new dimensions of health care in the hospital buildings. With the result, the role of biomedical equipment and the necessary engineering services in the hospital buildings have increased manifold. It has had a direct impact on the architectural planning of practically all-functional spaces in the building. In order to derive maximum advantage of technological advances, the planning of functional spaces needs to ensure that the engineering services are adequately and appropriately provided to facilitates proper utilization of equipment. This has been further complicated by the fact that each functional space may have more than one engineering service to be incorporated. It calls for a planning process of functional spaces wherein functional planning of health care is to be integrated with equipment and engineering service planning. For successful overall functional planning, a complete co-ordination is very essential.

In a planning process that has such high demands on co-ordination, it is imperative that the design brief and evolution of basic functional requirement is done in a manner that causes least changes to design of subsequent stages. Thus, the overall planning must ensure that each stage, functional requirements and anticipated performance of health care facilities reviewed by all the stakeholders. In essence, the nature of health care perceived and the facilities required should be planned at the pre-construction stage properly.

HOSPITAL CLASSIFICATION (Flow chart 3.1)

Hospital buildings can be classified in a variety of ways. In accordance with the nature of the health care provided, these buildings can be classified as primary, secondary and tertiary medical care facilities. This classification is in tune with the National Health Care Policy. A network of primary health care facilities supports upto 6 sub-centers or field units, catering to a population of about 100,000. Secondary health care facilities provide services to the patients referred from primary health care facilities. These are generally district level hospitals. Tertiary medical care provides superior level, super specialties include cardiac care, neuro-science facilities, etc. with necessary high-end diagnostic and laboratory support facilities. Depending upon the type of ownership, the hospitals include

Flow chart 3.1: Classification of hospital

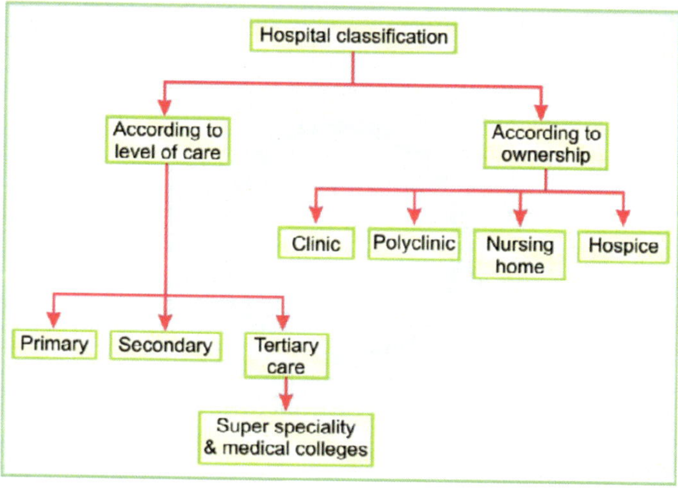

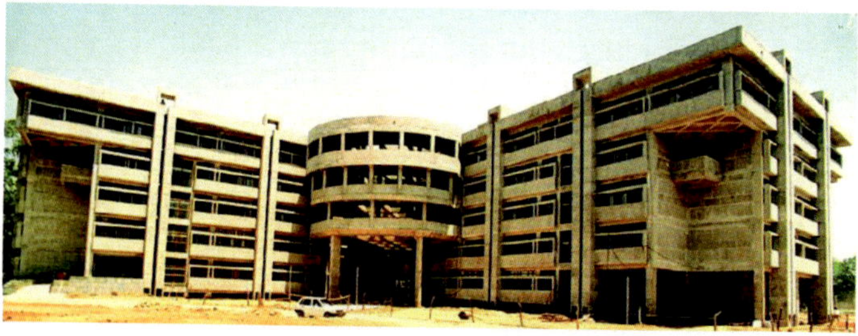

Fig. 3.1: Advanced Pediatric Centre, PGI Chandigarh; Arch. SD Sharma and Associates

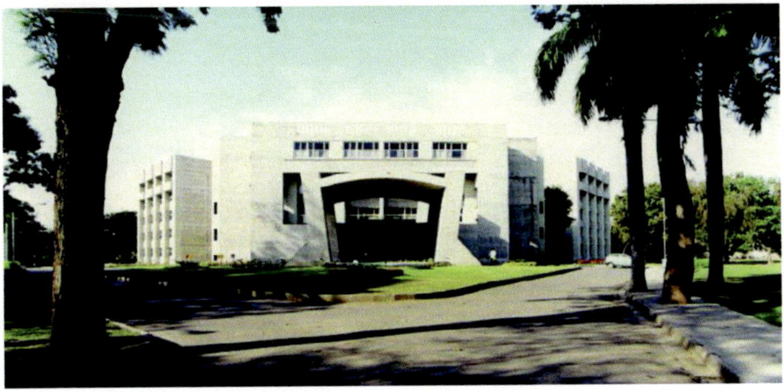

Fig. 3.2: OPD block at PGI Chandigarh; Arch. SD Sharma and Associates

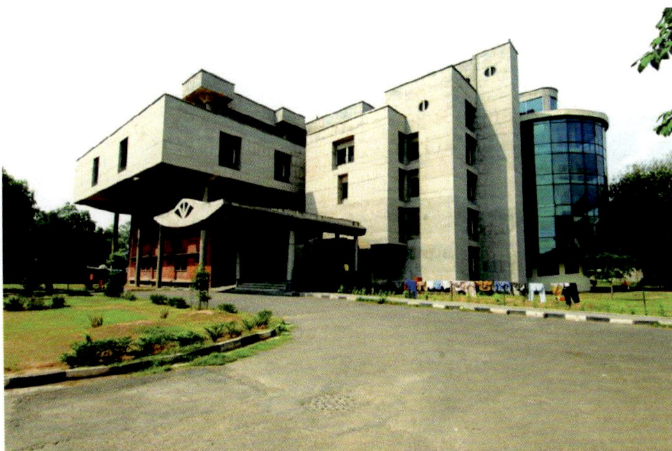

Fig. 3.3: Advanced Eye Care Centre at PGI, Chandigarh; Arch. SD Sharma and Associates

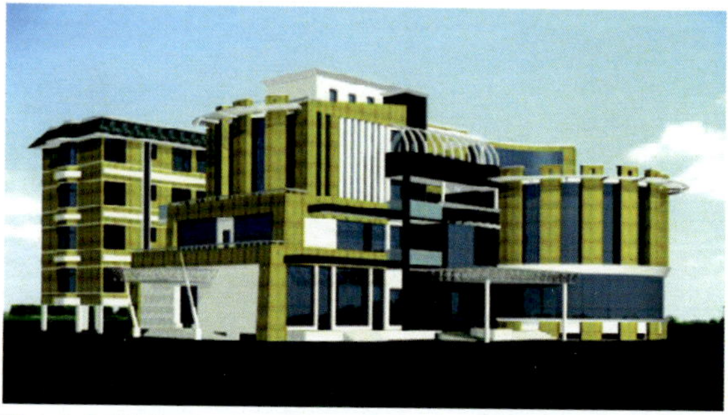

Fig. 3.4: Malhotra Hospital at Agra; Arch. Purnima Sharma

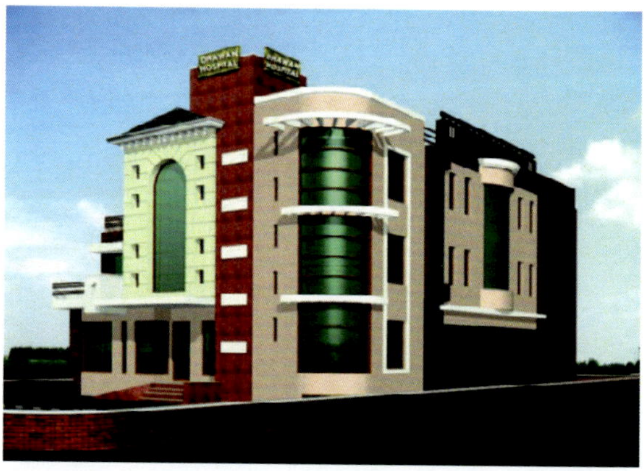

Fig. 3.5: Dhwan Hospital at Panchkula; Arch. Purnima Sharma

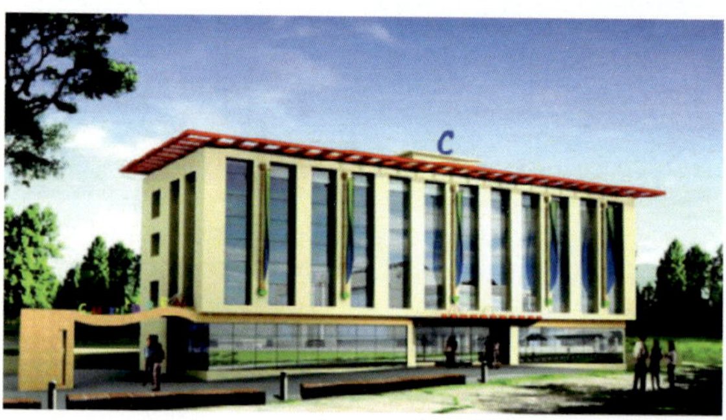

Fig. 3.6: KNS Children Hospital at Panchkula; Arch. Purnima Sharma

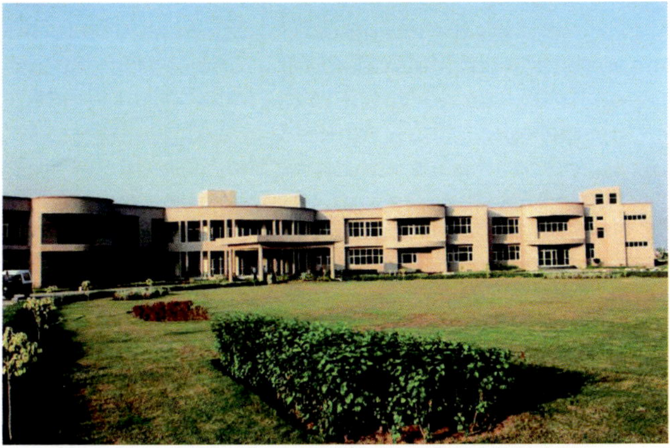

Fig. 3.7: Hospital for ordinance factory at Rajgir, Bihar; Arch. Sangeet Sharma

consultant clinics, polyclinics, nursing homes and hospice. Private hospitals could be owned by individual, trusts corporate sectors. In certain cases, joint venture with government institution/bodies is also resorted to. Indian standards provide functional planning norms for five categories of hospitals, A to E which range from 25-50 beds, 51-100 beds, 101- 300 beds, 301-500 beds, and 501-700 beds respectively. All teaching hospitals are required to have a minimum of 200 bed hospitals as a part of medical college. Such teaching hospitals are governed by the mandatory requirements established by the Medical Council of India.

PLANNING

ISSUE IN PLANNING OF HOSPITAL

Hospital building planning is directly related to the functional performance from the point of view of health care and the technological requirement to be fulfilled. The pace of 'technological advances has a tremendous impact on the future relevance of the facilities and high degree of obsolescence. Thus, while integrated planning of functional spaces in an issue, the future change is another aspect that has to be inherent in the planning though process. Structural systems of the buildings, architectural configuration, engineering services provisions (capacity and routing) and budgeting can complicate managerial decision and, if not considered properly, can lead to definite adverse impact on the quality of health care delivered by the hospitals. It can, thus, be concluded at this stage that pre-construction is the most critical phase of hospital building project. Involvement of all stakeholders in the pre-construction phased as a multidisciplinary team is one way to ensure that the planning is relevant.

REQUIREMENTS FOR PROPER HOSPITAL PLANNING (Flow chart 3.2)

Hospital requirements are worked out primarily through functional planning. Functional planning is the basis for incorporating other elements of building project, namely engineering services and equipment planning. For the purpose of hospital planning, various components/departments are taken into consideration. Each department is an independent entity and specific peculiarities. However, there are many interrelated aspects that need to be considered from the point of view of compatibility and supportive role. The broad categorization of various departments is as follows:

Flow chart 3.2: A proper hospital

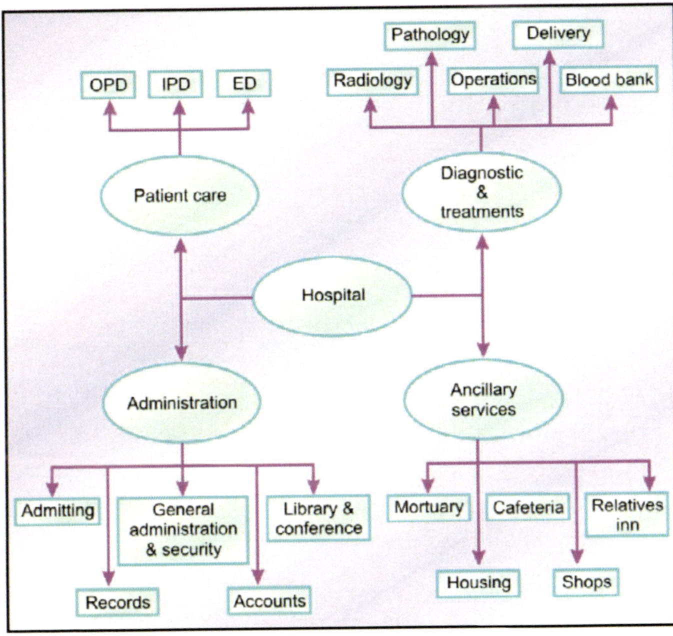

Patient Care Division

a. Outpatient department.
b. Inpatient department.
c. Emergency department.

Diagnostic and Treatment

a. Radiology.
b. Pathology.
c. Operation suites.
d. Delivery suites.

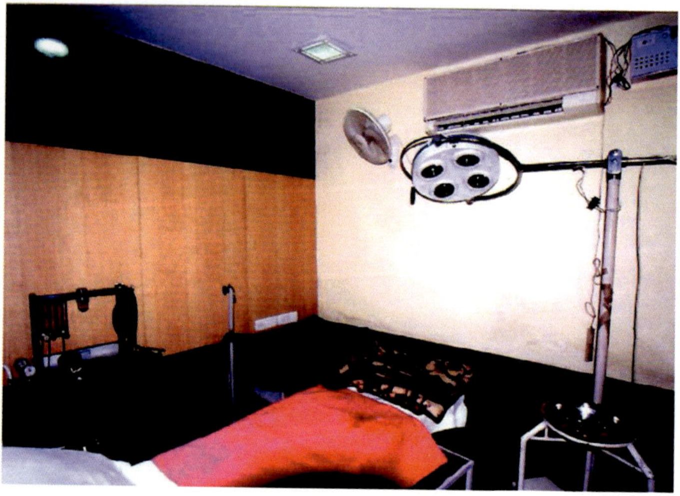

Fig. 3.8: Operation theater area

Administrative Service

a. Admitting.
b. Medical records.
c. General administration.
d. Accounts.
e. Library/conference.

Ancillary Services

a. Mortuary.
b. Housing.
c. Cafeteria.
d. Shops.
e. Relatives inn.

Inter-department and intra-departmental zoning is developed to ensure proper movement of hospital staff, doctors, patients and the service (especially clean and dirty services).

Flow chart 3.3: Hospital services

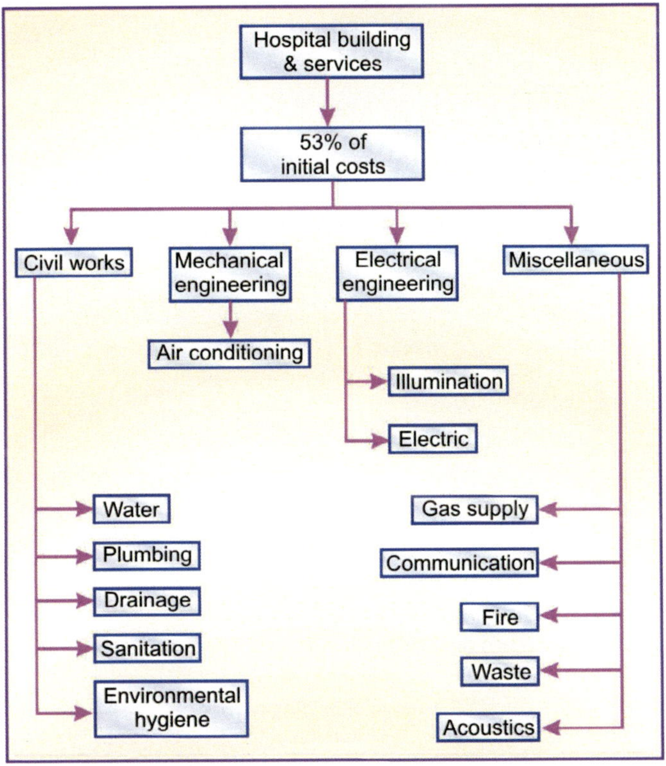

SERVICES PLANNING (Flow chart 3.3)

In the hospital building, the services contribute to about 53 percent of the initial capital cost. Operating and maintenance costs of the building are far more significant in case of services. The hospital planning should give equal importance to engineering service planning. Location and types of services are important since they are directly related to the functions of the building as per I.S. code, the engineering service requirement can be divided into the following sections:-

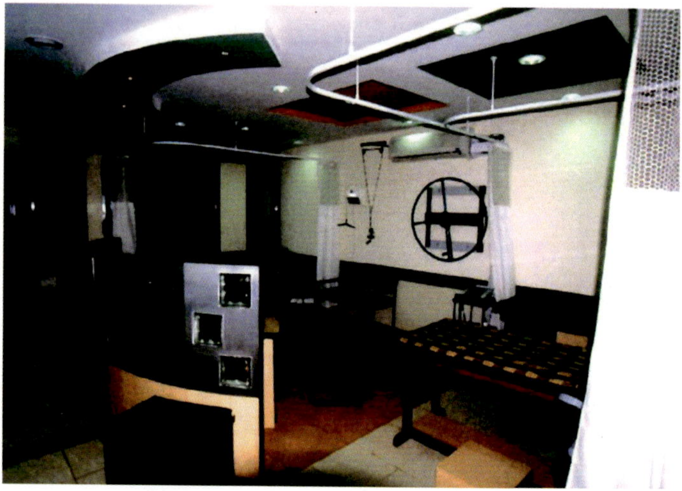

Fig. 3.9: Physiotherapy area of a clinic in Chandigarh

Civil

i. Water supply and plumbing
ii. Drainage and sanitation
iii. Environmental hygiene

Mechanical Engineering Department

i. Heating ventilation and air-conditioning

Electrical Engineering Department

i. Illumination
ii. Electric supply

Miscellaneous

i. Gas supply
ii. Communication

iii. Fire protection
iv. Waste disposal
v. Acoustics

INTEGRATION OF FUNCTIONAL AND SERVICE PLANNING

Integration of functional and service planning is important as it helps in identifying crucial stages in the installation. In certain cases installation of a particular service might have specific requirements with regards to process and structure, an integration of these would clearly bring prerequisites. For integration various interfaces are prepared and then accordingly the responsibilities are delegated to agencies. The integration not only highlights the inter-dependencies, but also their implications on the overall progress.

IDENTIFICATION AND PLANNING OF MEDICAL SERVICE AREAS

OPD AS ONE PROTOTYPE

Location

The OPD should ideally be on the ground floor, (in case of the hospitals of type C, D, E the numbers of clinics being more, it might need distribution between two or more floors. In such case it is recommended that surgical, orthopedics, antenatal, obstetric and gynecology and pediatric clinic are on the ground floor. Rest of the clinics can be placed on the upper floors preferably with the separate entrance and adequate parking facilities.

The reception area should be immediately apparent and welcoming on entering the department.

Table 3.1: Planning stages

Planning stages	*Team*	*Purpose/objective*
Preliminary evolution and concept stage	Client and consultant	The client in consultation with the consultant formulates project brief. This stage is basically framing of the requirements (functional and services). Analysis of the afore-mentioned leads to the preparation of the preliminary report.
Design stage	Client, consultant and hospital team	The consultant, well-integrated with the floor plans, as provided by the architect, prepares the detailed service plans. At times, there can be more than one service consultant preparing the service drawings.
Strategy planning	Client, consultant and hospital team	Based on the plans prepared, the strategy plan is prepared which includes the assignment of work within the organization and also the management integrated system.
Bidding stage	Consultant (architect + service consultant + project manager), client	Based on the plans (architectural and services), the work packages are decided and bids are invited from the contractors so that the work can be assigned to them.
Construction stage	Client, consultant (architect + project manager + service consultant), contractor	Construction takes place on the site.

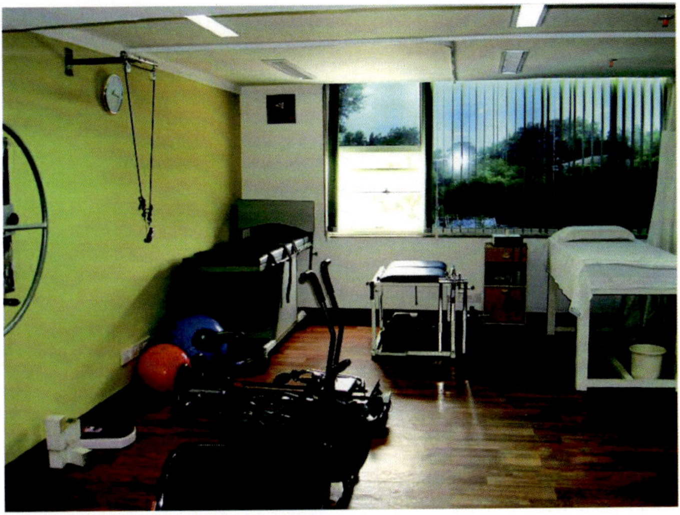

Fig. 3.10: Physiotherapy area

The reception point needs to adjoin the patient's record room; store and is sometimes combined with it.

It is worth noting that people who are unfamiliar with the building like to leave it by the same route from which they have entered and staff need a way in and out independent of that used by the patient.

Attention should be paid to circulation, which should result in the smooth flow of the various traffic lines traversing the department.

It should have easy access to the laboratories, radiology, pharmacy and the physical therapy departments since the patients use practically all the diagnostic and therapeutic department during every visit.

Each clinic should have its independent area, doctor's examination area and diagnostic/treatment area as required, e.g. surgical clinic shall have treatment-cum-dressing, and orthopedics clinic would have plaster preparation-cum-fracture treatment area, etc.

Treatment rooms for minor procedures and cast work should be easily accessible from the main waiting spaces and the consultation rooms.

DESIGN CONSIDERATION

- The storage areas for the wheelchairs and the stretchers should be neatly alcoved and should be away from the main traffic line, but at the same time should be easily accessible.
- The lobby and the lounge provide seating arrangement for the largest foreseeable number of people. A large number of people crowding in one single area creates an impression of cold impersonality and inefficiency.
- To improve that atmosphere, patients should be dispersed to the subsidiary or sub-waiting area adjacent/close vicinity to the clinics.
- Elevators easily accessible to the lobby are especially important for the cardiac and the obstetric patients who require immediate core in the respective areas.
- If the hospital has an outpatient surgery program, the ancillary rooms should be equipped for the minor surgeries not requiring the general anesthesia and for the general diagnostic procedures.
- A recovery room for holding the patients for observation after the surgery should be located adjacent to the minor surgery room. It should be visible from the nurse's station for supervision and observation.
- Other facilities that may be provided include the toilets, the place where the patients may change from the street clothes to the hospital gowns whenever necessary, the

space where they can keep their valuables, patients preparation area, the scrub and change rooms.

- There should be proper arrangement for keeping the major portion of the OPD locked after the outpatients hours.
- The linkage between the emergency services and the outpatient department for certain adjacent services such as medical records, etc. should be available to the staff and the emergency patients during the evening and night shifts.
- Registration cubicles designed to afford privacy and maintain patient's self esteem.
- Directional signs freely used throughout the department.
- Public areas with the provision for public telephones, patient's toilets, water coolers or drinking water fountains, inquiry counter desk, cashier booth, coffee shop/snack counter and if possible separate play areas for the children.
- The temperature requirement in the department, where controlled environment is required varies from 22 ±24°C. The rooms which require this kind of temperature level are:
  — Consultation rooms, examination rooms, observation rooms, ECG rooms, procedure room, sub-waiting, immunization room, social worker's room, minor O.T., seminar room. These rooms in the public hospital have the ambient temperature (temperature as per weather conditions, without the air being conditioned).
- The functional units such as stores, toilets, clean utility, dirty utility, janitor's closet, etc. can have ambient temperature.
- The relative humidity requirement in the departments, where controlled environment is required, varies from

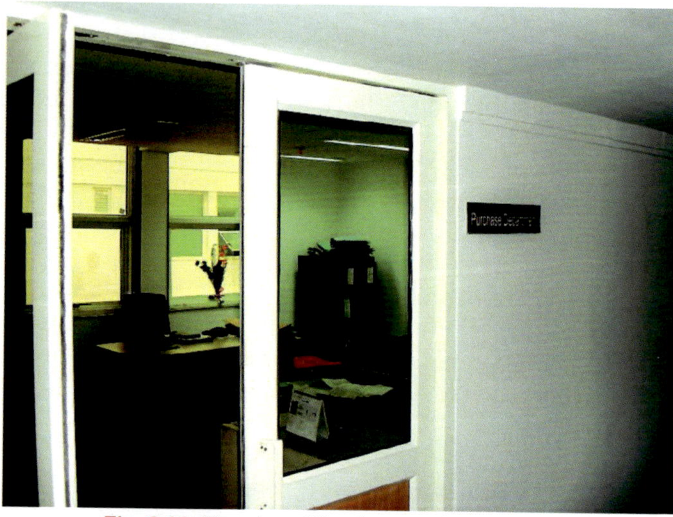

Fig. 3.11: The size of the doors and the top glass makes way for the visibility and control

55-60 percent. The rooms which require this kind of humidity level are:

— Consultation rooms, examination rooms, observation rooms, ECG rooms procedure room, sub-waiting, immunization room, social worker's room, minor O.T., seminar room. Rooms in the public hospital have the ambient temperature (humidity as per weather conditions without the air and moisture being conditioned).

- Functional units such as stores, toilets, clean utility, janitor's closet, etc. have ambient humidity level.
- The pressure in the functional units except for the clinical laboratories, dark room, toilets, janitor's closet, dirty utility where the pressure is kept negative (so that the air should not flow to the other spaces), is kept normal.

- The minimum air changes vary from 2 (almost all the functional units of the department) to 4 in the minor operating room in the general surgery room.
- The total air-changes may vary from 2 (in most of the functional units) to 4 in skin lab, denture lab, minor operating room (family planning), plaster cutting room, toilets, dirty utility, janitor's closet (procedure room, orthopedics operating room, general surgery operating room).
- The air from the skin lab, denture lab, minor operating room, plaster cutting room, toilets, janitor's closet and dirty utility has to be exhausted out and will not be re-circulated because the air, after the functions have been performed, has the bio-particulate material more than 350/cum (as against the clean air requirement which should have 0.5 micron particle upto 200/cum).

ELECTRIC AND ILLUMINATION SYSTEM

There are quite a few variations in the parameters of the functional units being catered by the electric and illumination part system and which are as under:

- The general illumination level in the hospital as the benchmark is taken as 150 lux.

The task illumination varies from:

- 150 lux (in consultation room, skin lab, sub-waiting, speech therapy room, observation room, denture lab, immunization room, reception and record, social worker's room, plaster cutting room, patient receiving room, etc.)
- 300 lux (in recovery room, treatment room, record room and cash counter, etc.)
- 500 lux in {in dental surgery (mouth), dental hygienist room, etc.

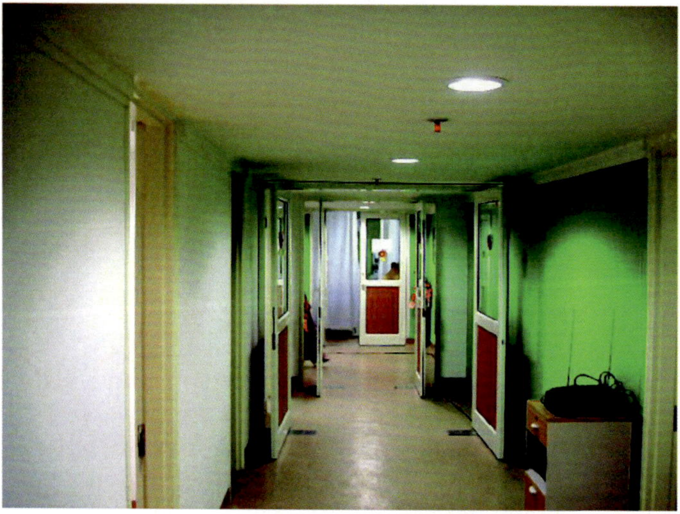

Fig. 3.12: The perfect illumination and ambience makes a difference for the patient

- 5000 lux in procedure room of obstetric and gynecological.
- 10000-40,000 lux (in dental surgery room).

The emergency task illumination varies from:

- 300 lux (in procedure room, recovery room, clinical laboratory, skin lab, seminar room, refraction room, dark room, etc.)
- 500 lux (in consultation room, audiometry room, denture lab, immunization room, recovery room, treatment room, etc.)
- 900 lux (in ECT room, minor operating room)
- There is a variation in the electric socket fixtures of 5, 15, 20 ampere. Depending upon the equipment used in the functional units.
- There are certain areas which require the stabilized power due to the equipment used in the functional unit

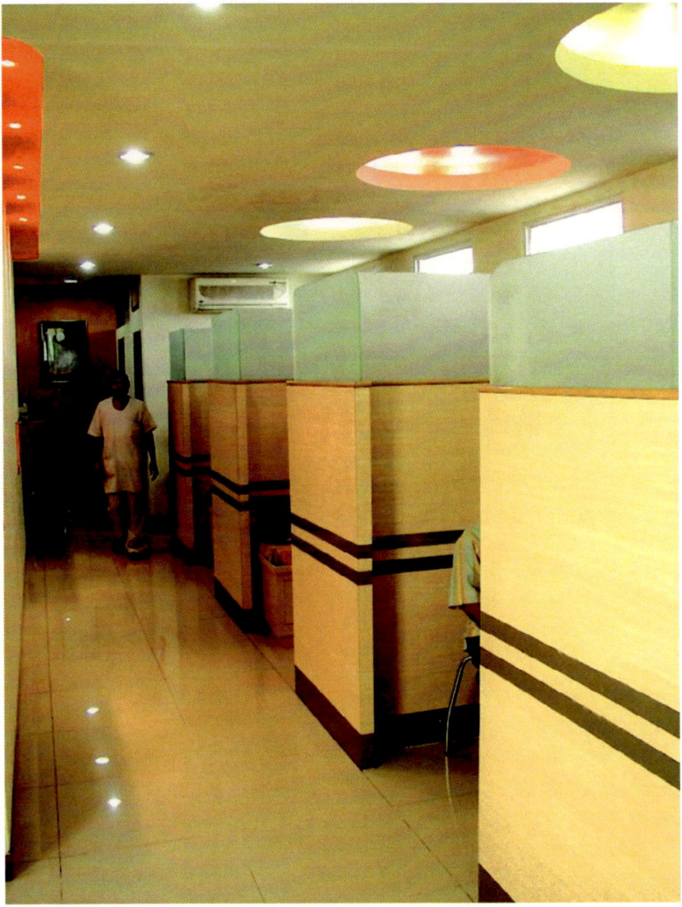

Fig. 3.13: Designer lighting and cabins at work

like (ECG room, speech therapy room, dental surgery, dental hygienist room, procedure room, plaster cutting room, minor operating room, seminar room, etc.), whereas there are certain areas which require constant

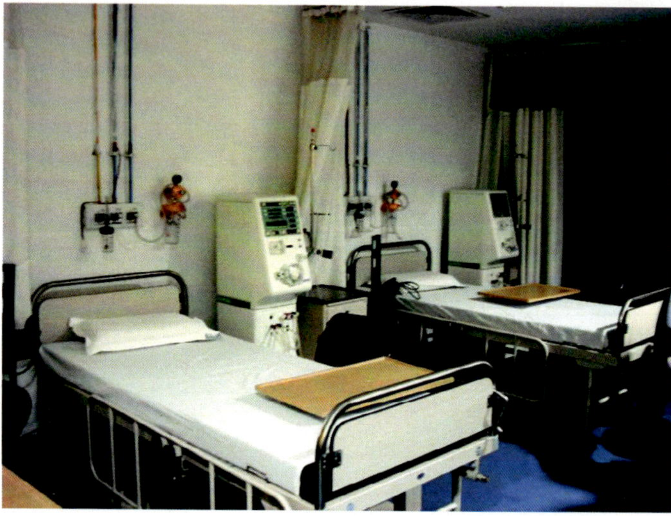

Fig. 3.14: The view of the ward area

supply of electricity as even the delay of few fraction of seconds may prove lethal like (minor operating room, ECT room, etc.).

SANITARY SYSTEM

There are quite a few variations in the parameters of the functional units being catered by the sanitary system and they are:

- The public address system is installed in the limited areas such as consultation rooms, OPD supervisor's office, OPD registration and reception counter where if at all some address is to be made in case of emergency, only the staff of the hospital comes to know about that, without creating the panic amongst the patients.

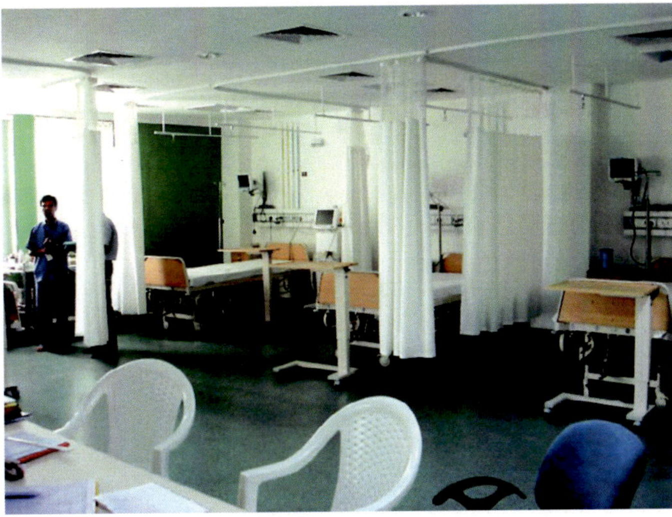

Fig. 3.15: ICU units

- The computer port if required in the audiometry room, recovery room, clinical laboratory, reception and record, orthopedics room, OPD reception area.
- The areas such as consultation room, minor operation room, social worker's room, dental surgery should have the provision for the computer port as in these areas the use can be optional.
- Washbasin with cold and hot water supply should be installed in the functional units such as consultation room with examination room, denture lab, dental surgery room, TB and chest clinic, skin lab, procedure room, recovery room, immunization room, sister's change room, etc. where the ablution facilities are required after the patient has been examined and diagnosed by the professional.

- The sink with the stone finish counter should be provided in the areas such as skin lab, denture lab, dental surgery room, procedure room, recovery room, clinical laboratory, minor operating room, plaster cutting room. The sink should be made of stainless steel and not concrete as the reagents and the chemical composition of the medicine lead to the hole formation in the concrete sink.
- The sink in the areas such as consultation room, examination room, social worker's room, sister's incharge's office may not be desirable and the provision there may be at the discrete decision of the hospital managing committee.
- The provision of steam in OPD areas is not desirable except for the denture lab.
- The floors of the areas such as skin lab, sub-room, speech therapy room and the recovery.

  The same analysis has been done for the other functional units of the hospital.

PMG ACOUSTICS AND FIRE DETECTION SYSTEMS

There are quite few variations in the parameters of the functional units being catered by the PMG acoustics and fire detection system and they are:

- The piped medical gases viz, oxygen, compressed air and vacuum are generally used, the nitrous oxide being used only for the anesthesia purpose in the surgical and obstetric suite.

HVAC and Illumination in Wards

- The minimum of 1000 mm of loft space should be left above the toilet space for the placement of FCU's. If the height is increased, the lumen intensity from the fixture is going to decrease, which means either the number of fixtures has to be increased or the fixtures with higher lumen output have to be used to meet the requirement of the ward.

HVAC and Water Supply

- Proper sleeves have to be left to allow the pipes to pass through (both chilled water supply and return). They too will run in the same shaft where other water supply and sanitation pipes run.

HVAC and Sanitation

- The drainage from the FCU to go through waste water pipe (in shaft with minimum 2 hour fire rating) which carries waste from washbasin, bath tub, etc.
- Proper sleeves have to be left to allow the pipes to pass through.

HVAC and Structure

- Structural members with the sleeves should be properly designed.
- Ceiling to be designed to support the equipment.
- The service penetration must be detailed to maintain acoustic and fire separation.
- The area where the functional equipment is placed{the loft and shaft (which houses the supply return and drainage pipes)} should provide easy accessibility for major alteration.

Illumination and Electric Supply

- Electric fixture should not cause any hindrance while the patient is lying on the bed. This implies that the position of the junction boxes for the placement of the electric fixtures shall be marked.

Illumination and Structure

- The fixtures, which require access for any reason should not be enclosed by structural component. The service distribution lines and terminals shall be surface mounted.

ELECTRIC SUPPLY AND STRUCTURE

- Structure should provide adequate support and efficient passage for electric cables.

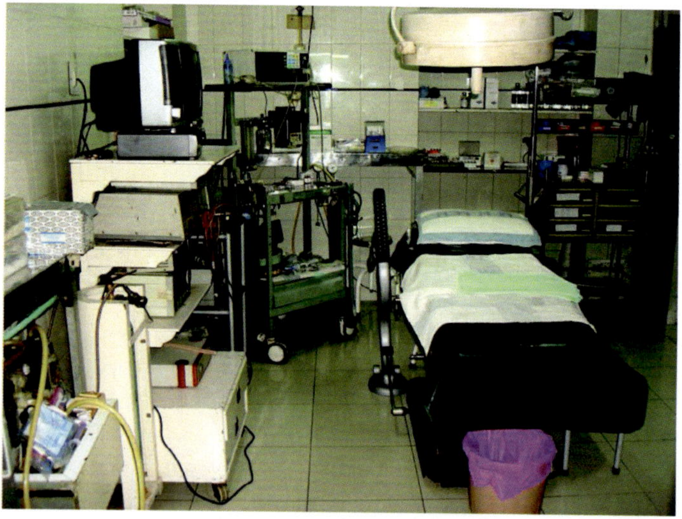

Fig. 3.16: The typical operation theater and its paraphernalia

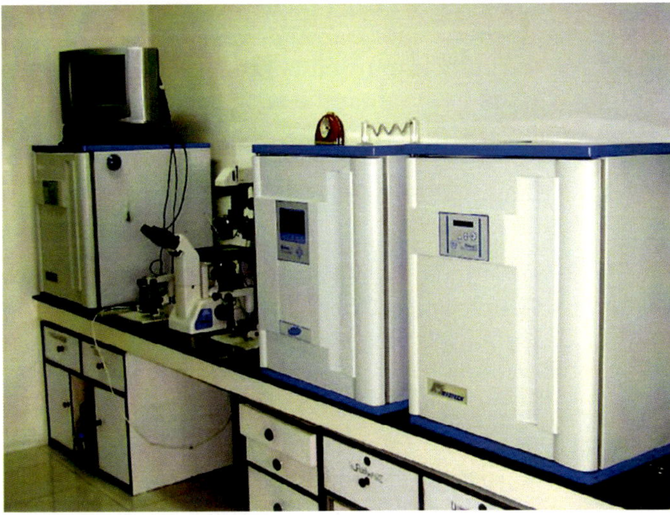

Fig. 3.17: Specialized services and equipments (I.V.F. Lab.)

- Service penetration should be detailed out to maintain acoustic and fire separation.
- Due consideration should be given to the filling material (partitions) as it is on these surfaces that the electric conduits run vertically.

WATER SUPPLY AND SANITATION

The position of the sanitary fixtures (ideally the principle of dry, semi-dry and wet should be followed) will affect the layout of the water supply (hot/cold and the returns for the same) and sanitary pipes, which instead can be the restriction on the location of the partitions under that very floor.

- Proper care should be taken that these pipes do not cross or overlap each other.

- The used water from the bath area and the washbasin through the floor trap and waste water pipe should go to the gully trap from where it finally go to the sewer.
- The soil waste from the wc goes to the sewer through soil waste pipe.

WATER SUPPLY AND STRUCTURE

- The restriction on the service drops locations can affect the location of partitions, fixtures and equipment.
- Adequate access door to the interior of the shaft should be provided for the purpose of maintenance and alterations.

SANITATION AND STRUCTURE

- Gravity drains are the only component of the service distribution, which feed through the floor. Therefore, the structure should provide adequate and efficient passage of all components in a manner so as to cause least possible restriction on the location of drains.
- The service drops of sanitary pipes should not corner in the areas such as operation theaters, ICU, ICCU, etc.
- Adequate access (door) to the interior of the shaft should be provided for the purpose of maintenance and alterations.
- The sanitary fixtures shall be fitted on the site once the flooring and initial coats of white washing have been done.

CONCLUSION

Service in health care facilities are quite complex and are dependent on the peculiarities of the function for which the various functional units are designed. There persists a

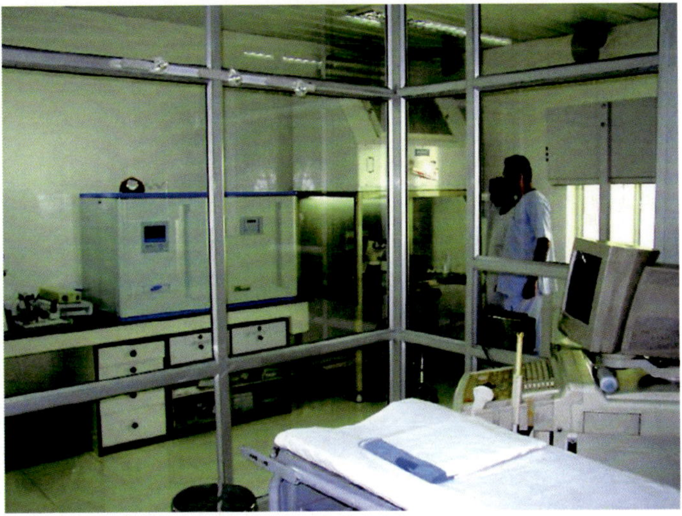

Fig. 3.18: A view of typical IVF unit

lack of awareness and consciousness regarding these, amongst the so-called professionals associated with the health facilities. It is imperative that the issue of the uncertainties is addressed through a well-defined system. Early identification of uncertainties, and issue of defects and method of timely control will enhance the effectiveness and efficiency of the construction.

SERVICES

Engineering Services

As explained earlier, practically all engineering services needed in the operation theater department would be needed here in toto. At present, patient monitoring is not widely employed but with latest development it may get

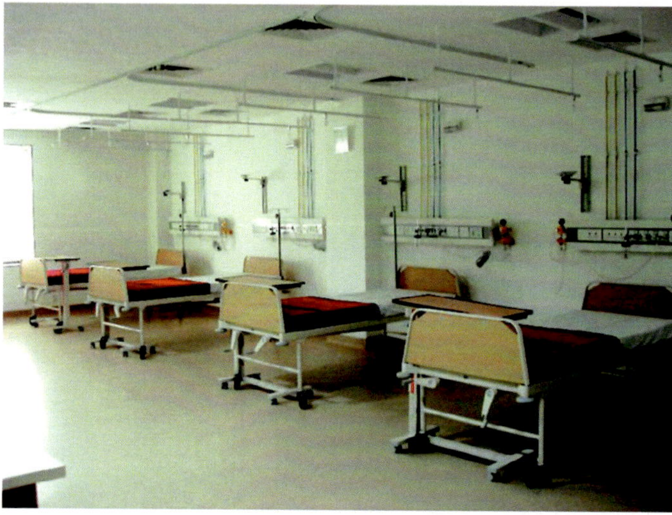

Fig. 3.19: The management of services is an important area for the planning

introduced very soon. For this purpose, necessary conduits and wiring provisions should be made in patients as well as nurses area in advance.

SPECIFICATIONS

For clean, hygienic and sound control conditions, floor and dado to sill heights should be of resilient material, such as marble. Walls should have plastic emulsion or washable oil-plastic emulsion or washable oil-bound distemper finish and joinery shall also be painted with plastic emulsion paints. Precautions should be taken against explosion hazards and electric fittings sparks in this unit.

Certain fixtures and special fittings, such as overhead curtain rails for screening off the beds, extra-electric outlets with each bed and heavy deity electric outlets per subunit, central piped suction gases and fuel gas, elbow/knee operated sinks in patients, nurses and clean utility areas should be provided. X-ray viewing boxes flush to wall in nurses and MO's duty room and double leafed winder doors to patients are major necessities of the unit.

SPECIFICATION, ESSENTIAL FITTINGS AND FIXTURES IN HOSPITALS

Cast *in situ* flooring should be provided where washing is frequent, otherwise tiles would suffice. Terrazzo, in general, is authorized instead of marble to reduce noise due to walking or falling of instrument. In radiography room, the floor has to be of insulating material like rubber or wood. In gymnasium too, wood floor is preferable for routine exercise and rehabilitation needs. In chemical lab, acid resisting tiles should be used in flooring.

Skirting and Dado

To maintain cleanliness and to provide protection against damage to walls by movement of trolleys dado is advisable in wards and corridors besides areas where dado is a must. For lab, toilets, kitchens and surgery, laboratories and dispensary the dado needs to be of glazed tiles to avoid sticking of greasy matter on the surface.

All over skirting and dado should be made flush to wall surface to avoid collection of dust.

Walls and Ceiling

Use of washable distemper or emulsion paint in general is, permitted to maintain hygienic cleanliness. Color wash or white wash is given to room/areas where there is no activity of patients hospitalization. In the operation threater, walls must be fully terrazzo finished.

For sound proofing of audiometry room, insulation should be done by the use of glass wool, cork or insulation boards. Aluminium paint for ultraviolet room in physiotherapy, acid and alcoholic proof wall for film developing dark room and lead lining to protect against radiation in superficial X-ray therapy are special requirements.

There should not be any projection as a place for dust collection. For this, as far as possible fittings and fixtures should be made flush to the wall surface. All wiring should be concealed.

Joinery

Flush shuttered wooden doors and steel or aluminium windows in general should be provided. Lead lined door in radiography, insulated steel air tight door for cool room and cold storage, venetian blinds to control glare in eye department/ward and fly proofing to doors and windows in infectious diseases ward, dining rooms, ward kitchen and server, animal houses, canteen and fresh ration supply stores are some special requirements.

Glazing of windows should be done with sheet glass, but for specific purposes special type of glass, such as frosted or fluted glass for toilets and lavatories, insulating type for sound proof rooms, colored glass for dark rooms and heat absorbing glass for air conditioned rooms, satin finish glass in operation theaters should be provided.

Hospitals are the most service-intensive buildings and so they merit a lot of though at the design level. Integration of basic building services like electrical, plumbing/ sanitary, air-conditioning ventilation and fire protection services in architecture design of hospitals is the basic need of today.

The first part of this paper can be used by architects as a planning tool, second part can be utilized as an understanding of design consideration made by a services design consultant.

VARIOUS FEATURES ARE DIVIDED UNDER FOLLOWING SUBHEADS

- Difference in hospital air-conditioning from comfort air-conditioning.
- Major areas in the hospital based on distinct services requirement.
- Identification of services required in a hospital design.
- Impact of architectural design on services design.
- Impact of site location, locality available resources and their conservation regulations.

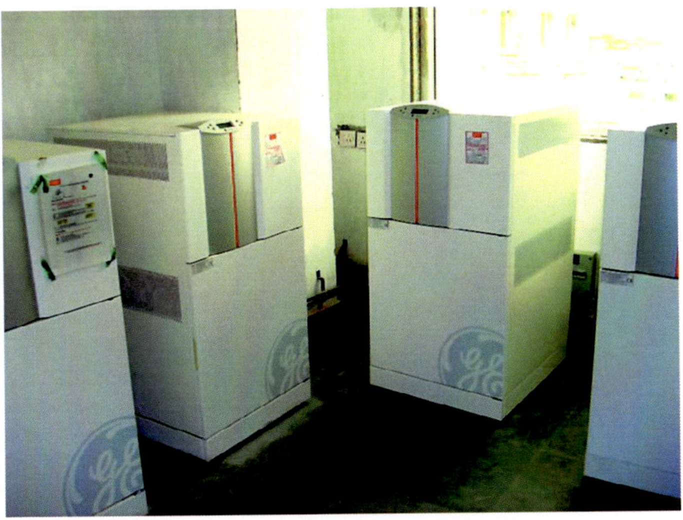

Fig. 3.20: Backup battery power supply

- Impact of regulations
- Impact of new technologies from an efficient building point of view
- Services design criteria from the maintenance point of view
- Fire risk in a hospital
- Contractors and administrative issues
- General issues in a hospital design from energy conservation point of view
- Operation theater design consideration
- Sterilization design consideration
- Maintenance problems faced due to improper architectural design considerations
- Vaastu consideration.

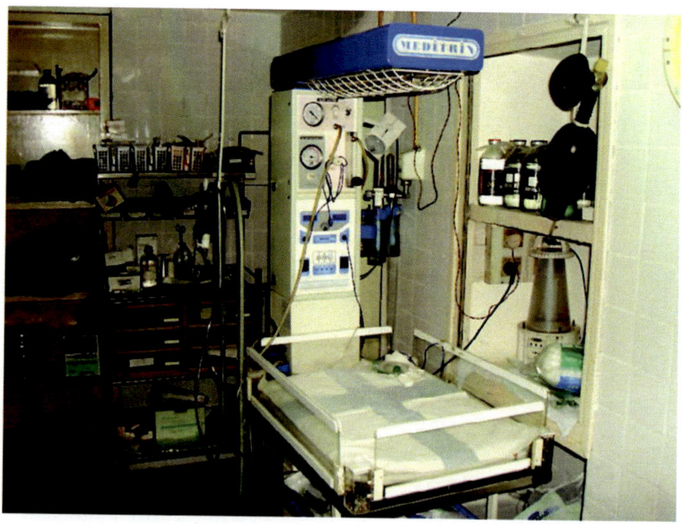

Fig. 3.21: The cable management is another except of detailing

Difference in Hospital Air-conditioning from Comfort Air-conditioning

The basic difference between air-conditioning for hospitals and for other building types are as follows:

Hospital air-conditioning assumes a more important role towards patients than the promotion of comfort. In many cases, proper air-conditioning is a factor in the therapy of the patient and in some instances, it is the major treatment. For example, cardiac patients and patients who are subjected to brain operations need environment in which the patient can lose heat by radiation and evaporation. It needs cooled and dehumidified air which requires dry bulb temperature of 68 ± 2°F (20°C ± 1°C) and RH 50 ± 5 percent.

Dry environment of 90° (32.2°C) and 35 percent RH has been used over an extended period for treatment of patients with rheumatoid arthritis.

Burn patients require 90°F (32.2°C) and RH upto 95 percent.

The need to restrict air movement in and between the various departments, i.e. air movement should be from clean to less clean area.

Ventilation and filtration to dilute/remove contamination in the form of odour and air-borne micro-organisms.

The need for accurate control of environmental condition in various areas.

Major Areas in the Hospital Based in Distinct Services Requirements

The following areas represent a hospital on a component level. These areas have been identified based on their services need. The list is not exhaustive and limited to the following but may vary from hospital to hospital.

a. ICU (Intensive Care Unit) and CCU (Critical Care Unit).
b. OT and Sterile zone.
c. Nuclear medicine.
d. Laundry.
e. CSSD (Central Sterile Supply Department).
f. Kitchen and cold storages.
g. Labs.
h. Mortuary.
i. HVAC plant room.
j. AHU rooms.
k. Electrical substation.
l. Generator rooms and electrical panel room.
m. Boiler rooms.
n. Gas manifolds (hospital gases).
o. LPG gas banks.
p. Fuel storage.
q. Incinerator.

Thumb Rules and Other Design Considerations

a. As a general thumb rule a minimum of 8 to 10 percent of total floor area is required for services.
b. One ton of refrigeration is required for 150 to 180 sq.ft. of conditioned area, for all special areas like OTs where 100 percent fresh air is required, the system TR capacity is worked out separately.
c. An Air Handling Unit room preferably should be of size 4 m × 3.5 m × 2.5 m height.
d. A minimum height of about 4.5 < below soffit of beam is required for plant rooms consisting of DG sets, chillers and panels.
e. Plumbing shafts should be planned vertically and all shafts should terminate at terrace and not in between the floor.

f. Shafts should have enough space for the service personal to access and work for maintenance after installation.
g. Electrical room and electrical shaft should preferably be in one vertical stack, which optimizes the cost of electrical cables including line losses and minimizes the maintenance.
h. Water conservation—use of water in various posh colonies in New Delhi.
i. Fuel storage and gas banks are physically separated from the main building.
j. Effect of change in climate global warming.

Identification of Services Required in a Hospital Design

a. HVAC system design as per area/space requirement.
b. Gas supply (medical gases and LPG).

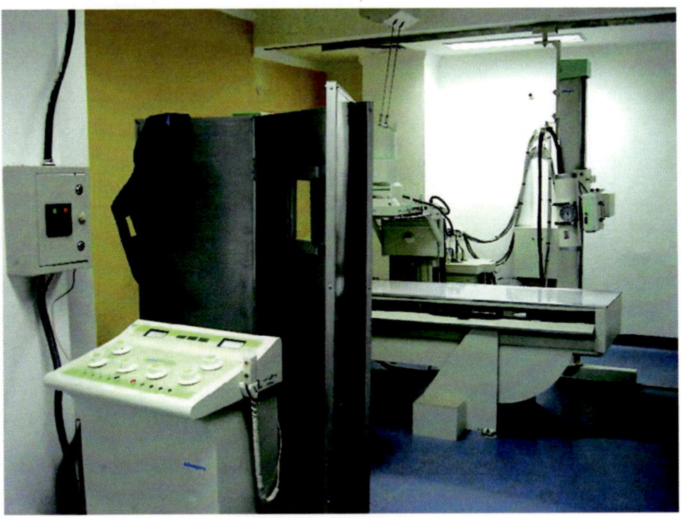

Fig. 3.22: The clean environment of X-ray unit

c. Boilers and steam generators.
d. Electrical system.
e. Fire detection and fighting (intelligent/conventional).
f. Sanitation and public health engineering including effluent/sewage treatment plant for recycling of treated effluent for gardening and make-up of cooling towers.
g. Water supply system (hot water and cold water supply, landscaping pumps, filtration plant, etc.).
h. Security system and data cable networking for computers, telephone data communication.
i. Pollution control for air and water pollution.
j. Refuse and garbage (organic, non-organic, solid waste) management.
k. Specific departmental needs like:
   - RO plant for ICU and dialysis, etc.
   - Blood washing
   - Bedpan wash

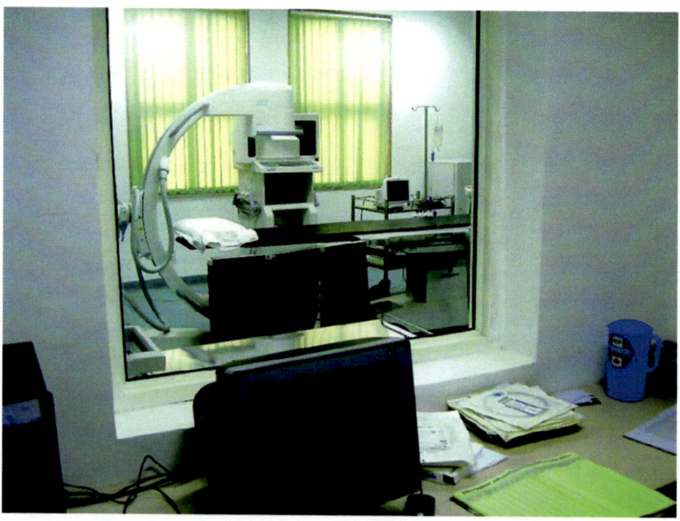

Fig. 3.23: The glass pane is perfect for monitoring

- Separation of infected/biohazard from normal sewage.

Impact of Architectural Design on Services Design

a. Increase in architectural use of glass in terms of structural glazing increases the HVAC load. The running cost becomes high and at the later stage HVAC design is questioned. Architects should do proper orientation study and take inputs about services cost right from day one of planning.
b. False ceiling material is important as it can help contain or accelerate contamination in terms of allergic reactions to fibers, fungus, bacteria and pest, etc.
c. False ceiling should also have the ability to endure condensation. In a few cases the condensation from HVAC pipes have caused the POP ceiling to get wet and even moulds formation.
d. Roof insulation has an impact on the running cost and overall heat load of the building.
e. Floor should be impervious and must be of anti-static composition.

Impact of Regulations

a. *Hospital design:* National Building Code Local Bye-laws and National Environmental Pollution Rules and Regulation.
b. *Nuclear medicine:* BARC approval, specific attention to prevent radioactive material from contaminating the main sewage system.
c. *Laundry and CSSD:* Electrical, fire codes, sanitation and plumbing codes.
d. *Mortuary:* Safety, PHE and hospital administrative policies and regulations.

e. *Electrical panel room and substation:* Electrical, fire and safety codes as per Indian Electricity Rules.
f. *Generator rooms:* DG sets recommendations, electrical, fire and pollution codes.
g. *Boiler rooms:* Boiler codes recommendations, electrical and fire regulations.
h. Availability and conservation of water has become a major issue as there is continuous depletion of underground water table which is of serious concern. Approval is required from Ground Water Authority for new bare wells. Contamination of ground water has been a major concern. The contaminated water becomes a matter of litigation and is a serious threat to public health.

Impact of New Technologies from an Efficient Building Point of View

IBMS

Intelligent Building Management System can give live data and reports; operators can use these data and refine the operation to suit their needs. Considerable energy savings can be achieved using IBMS. Security can also be integrated into this system. The automations can generate enough data to check system performance review and plan maintenance accordingly.

Services Design Criteria (mostly HVAC Design) from Maintenance Point of View

Air Intake and Exhaust Discharge Points

The design and locations of air intakes and exhaust discharge points play very important role in architectural

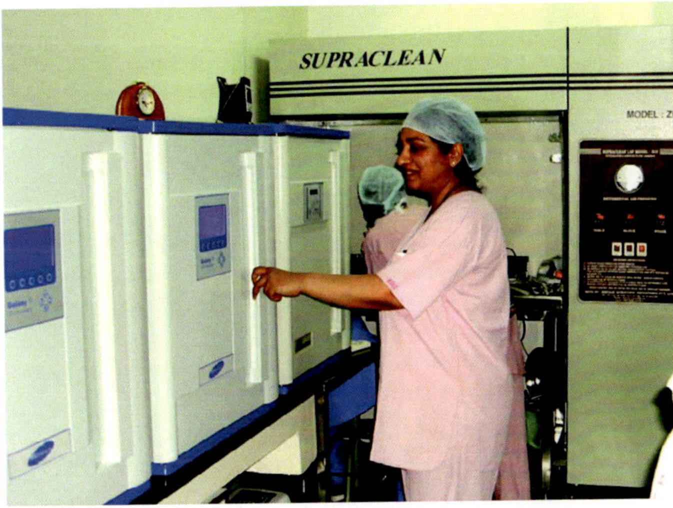

Fig. 3.24: Cleanliness, efficient planning and space management in Dr Jaideep Malhotra's IVF Center of MNMH Agra

design. Exhaust air effluents containing chemical or other pollutants coming from fume hoods, emergency generators, OT's exhausts should not short circuit with fresh air intakes.

Metal Deterioration from Moisture/Condensate

a. No fibrous material is allowed to be in contact with the airstreams in duct and plenum linings, including above ceiling return air plenums.
b. Drip pans need to be stainless steel and the design needs to address water carried by air as well as preventing water from flooding in the pans.
c. Trapped drains need to be located in the AHU room.

d. Sound attenuation devices exposed to high moisture conditions such as air humidifiers or cooling coil condensation must maintain their integrity for the life of the system.

Fire Risk in a Hospital

a. Hospitals are supposed to perform at 100 percent efficiency in case of emergency and disasters. In modern architectural practice, hospitals are closed glass boxes. A proper fire planning is an absolute must. Architects must see and refer to the fire codes as an important planning tool.
b. Now latest equipment is available for fire detection and suppression. These devices can instantly detect smoke and fire and appropriate alarms can be triggered identifying the exact zone/location of fire. Increased use of electronic storage equipment and imaging department needs specialized fire fighting equipment. The electrical areas have their own sets of requirements.
c. Regular fire drills/checks and training of fire personnel are required to ensure smooth operability of each fire protection equipment during emergency.

Contracts and Administrative Issues

a. Time of appointment of services consultant is also an issue. Usually the architects have a tendency to appoint consultants when the majority of design decisions have already been taken. So there may be constraints in accepting changes suggested by consultants.
b. Care must be taken to avoid architectural charges after the services contracts have been awarded. At times during execution of the contract, it is noticed that

architectural designs are changed very frequently after the services contracts have been issued. This leads to major problems in terms of equipment performance, services designs and project cost over run.

General Issues in a Hospital Design from Energy Conservation Point of View

a. Main load feeding center (DG Sets and Main LT Panel) shall be closer to Air-conditioning Plant, Water supply and Fire Pumps to minimize the capital cost of cables and line losses.
b. Electrical/Mechanical plant room (Utility Block) area should either be housed in a separate building or in the lower (second) basement to minimize noise of DG sets and A/c plant from transferring to public/patient's areas.
c. Locate underground water storage tank considering location of bore well, municipal line connection or tanker connection.
d. Under deck or over deck roof insulation of conserve energy and minimum use of heat and noise transfer, preferably cavity walls with sandwiched insulation may be considered.
e. Incandescent lamps shall be replaced with CFL lamps to conserve energy.
f. Increase the vegetative cover from environmental considerations.

Operation Theater Design Consideration

a. The operation theater should have walls and floor of impervious semi-matt surface with antistatic flooring. Tiles are not recommended due to crevices formed between each.

b. Ducting material should be aluminium. Care must be taken during duct fabrication and joints must be properly sealed to avoid any collection of dust particles/growth of bacteria.
c. It is preferred to have "laminar flow", in the OT's. The air coming out from 'Laminar flow diffusers' in the OT's passing through the efficient filters to remove inherent contaminations. The exhaust shall be taken through lower level extract grilles.
d. 20 to 30 air changes in the operation theater reduce the incidence of contamination.
e. There should be horizontal and vertical separation in fresh air intake and exhaust of OTs.
f. It is preferred to have separate AGU for each OT so that flexibility in terms of fumigation and control of temperature as per individual OT requirement can be maintained.
g. It is advisable to have a heating coil in the OT's AHU for RH (Relative humidity) and temperature control.
h. OT's AHU should maintain degree of pressurization so that the air should leak away to the other areas.

Sterilization Design Consideration

a. Instruments can be sterilized by steam, utilizing a portable autoclave or pressure type cooker. The sterilized equipment is supplied from:
   HSDU—Hospital Sterilizing and Disinfective Unit.
   CSSD—Central Sterile Supply Department.
   TSSU—Theater Sterile Supply Unit.
b. Air handling duct system shall be designed with accessibility for duct cleaning.
c. Care should be taken to avoid any water logging in AHU drain to avoid any growth of molds.
d. Provision should be made in AHU for housing the fumigators to fumigate during fumigation.

Problems Faced Due to Poor Design Consideration

1. Usually the fresh air and extract air gets mixed up as they both happen on the roof. Poor architectural space allocation is the cause of it.
2. The Gensets emission also has to be separated from the space/area from where fresh air is being taken in.

Often it has been observed that adequate space is not made available for routing of ducts, pipe-lines, cables and proper room for locating electrical panels and AHUS. Usually the planners treat this space as a Non-paying space. So they make it small and tight from maintenance point of view.

Chapter 4

Planning and Design Consideration for OT Block and ICU

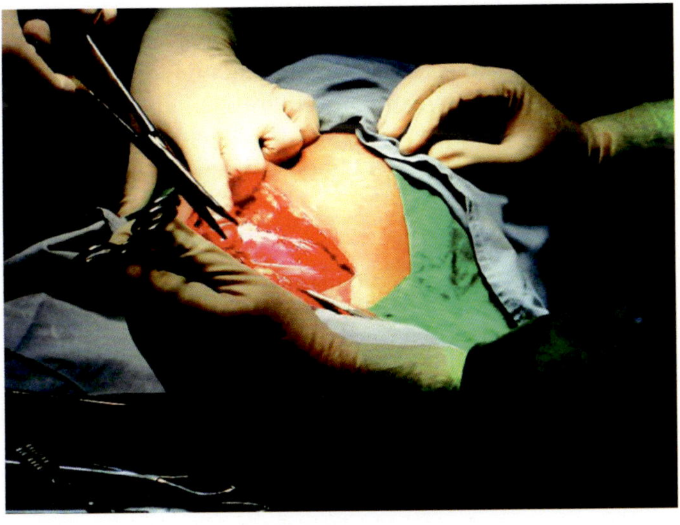

An operation in progress.

OPERATION THEATER CONCEPT

PREAMBLE

The operating department is the most important surgical facility provided in any hospital complex. Herein the clinical needs and requirements reach a point of real complexity. Considerations of requirements of staff, the patients and the overall bacteriological control to achieve the highest degree of aspects have a direct bearing on planning, circulation and the equipment to be provided.

LOCATION

Location of the OT block in the overall layout needs a critical study (Flow chart 4.1). The factors to be borne in mind are (i) quiet environment (ii) freedom from noise and other disturbances (iii) freedom from contamination and possible cross-infection (iv) good natural light orientation

Flow chart 4.1: Operation theater concept

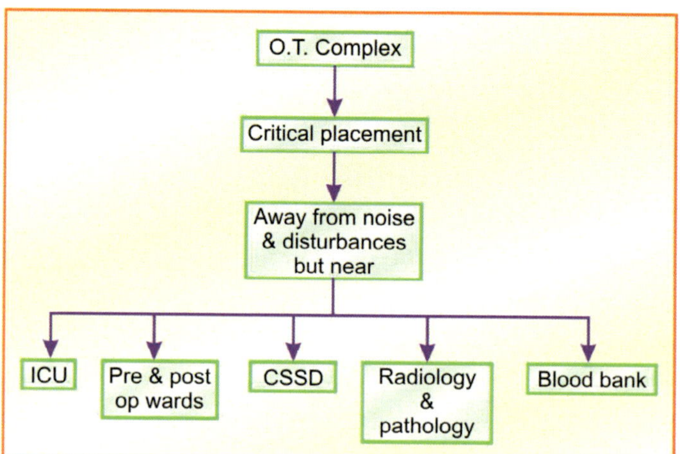

Flow chart 4.2: The planning approach and people involved

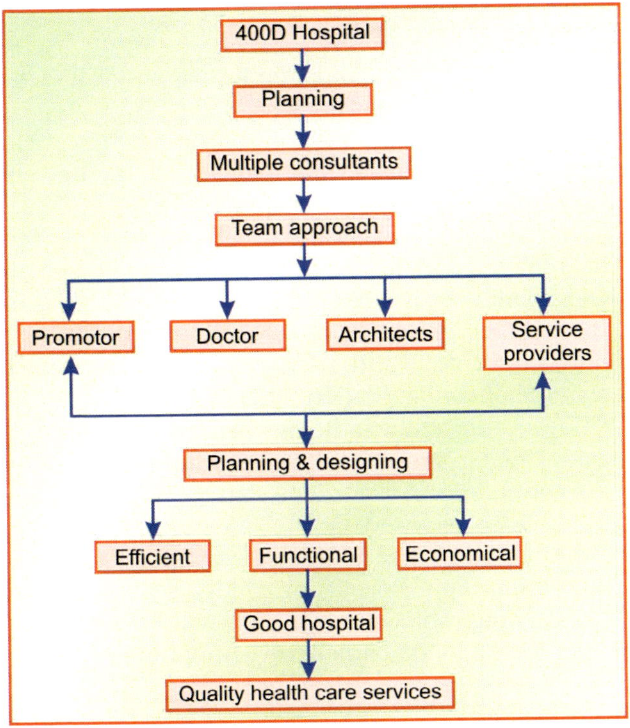

and (v) correct and convenient relationship with surgical ward, ICU, X-ray, pathology lab, etc.

The above three considerations stress the need for an elevated location in a detached block preferable on the topmost floor conveniently grouped with other facilities so as to cut down noise and unwanted movements of men and material.

The OTs can have a viewing gallery on top in a teaching hospital/specialist hospital.

RELATIONSHIP WITH OTHER DEPARTMENT AND WARDS

OT being obviously the most important surgical facility. The following provisions are necessary:

a. It should be closely linked with the intensive care unit and surgical wards, particularly the acute/post-operative.
b. This being the major user of CSSD, its location should be in the vicinity for the CSSD.
c. Close link with ICU which also provides the ultimate in medicare is important for optimum utilization of both equipment and specialist staff, lessening the chances of contamination/infection.
d. Close location of the radiology department is desirable, as during operation a quick check-up or consultation may be necessary; in addition staff to operate or process films, etc. is required.
e. Para pathological tests connected with operations are very important; hence its proximity is also desirable.
f. Often enough blood transfusion will be necessity; so close link of blood bank is very important.

ORIENTATION

The requirement for an operation theater is to have adequate glore-free natural light which has a germicidal psychological impact and hence north light is desirable. In addition, proper orientation reduces the heat gain with reference to the airconditioning load. It is true that most of the present day operations are performed under artificial light, but due to above considerations, good light and ventilation are of added advantage. This is also important in the case of any breakdown and during cleaning activities after the operation is over.

MAIN PLANNING CONSIDERATIONS

The basic aim would be to achieve the maximum level of sterility with streamlined circulation of traffic movements. The factors to be considered are:

a. Clean and dirty traffic streams be segregated.
b. The department should be independent of general traffic movement from the rest of the hospital.
c. Subzoning to produce successively higher degree of sterility with actual OT as the completely sterile zone.
d. Staff, patients, entry and exits to be segregated. This will streamline the circulation pattern.
e. Dirty material to be removed without passing through the clean zone.

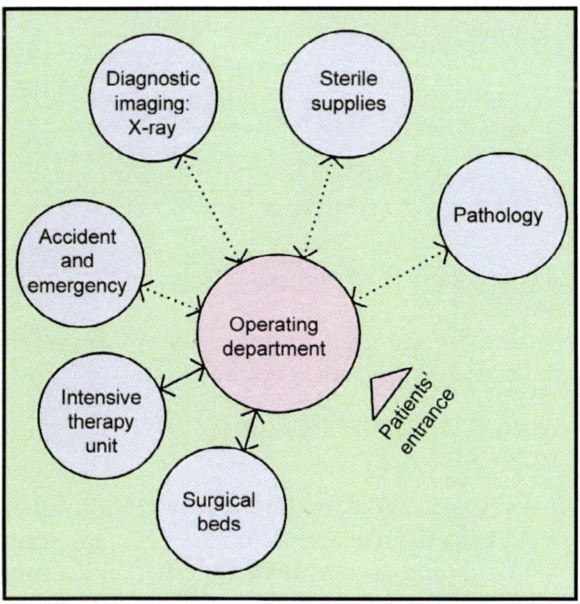

Fig. 4.1: Planning of emergency and sterile areas

Flow chart 4.3: Typical operation theater

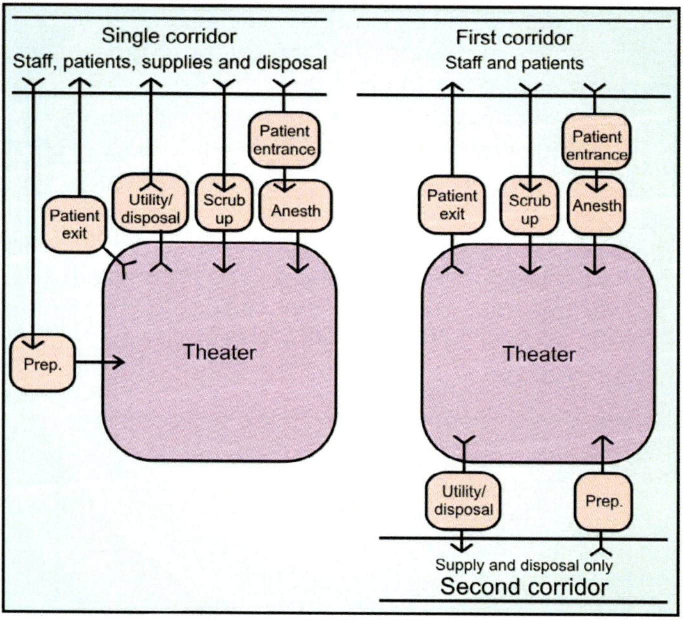

f. Direction of air-flow should be from clean to unclean zone.
g. Provision of comfortable climatic conditions, amenities to patients and staff for work and rest.

PLANNING STRATEGY BUILDING UP OF A CONCEPT

The ideal sitting is in the top floor of a hospital, as the area is free from bacterial contamination. As a general principle, all theaters should be grouped together in an integral whole, so as to be independent of air movement in the rest

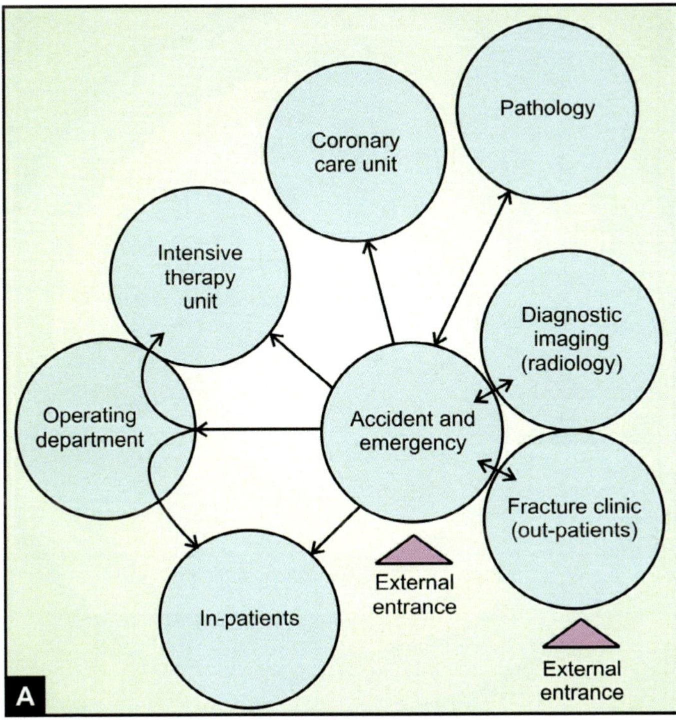

Fig. 4.2A

of the hospital, thus concentrating while programming surgical work.

It simplifies supply and disposal arrangement and allows full utilization with economy in staff use and services. Space utilization is further achieved by centralizing common ancillaries and providing of a central recovery unit.

The operation theater and ancillaries are so grouped that a proper progression of sterility is achieved and the

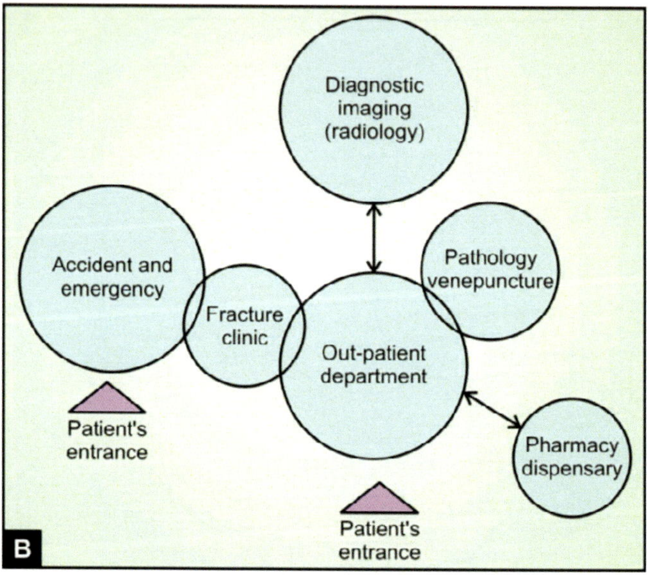

Figs 4.2A and B: Typical planning

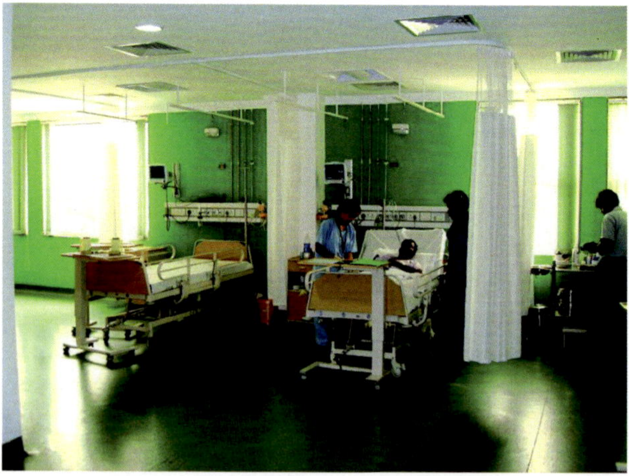

Fig. 4.3: All the factors of planning, services, colors and spaces play an important role for the healing of the patient

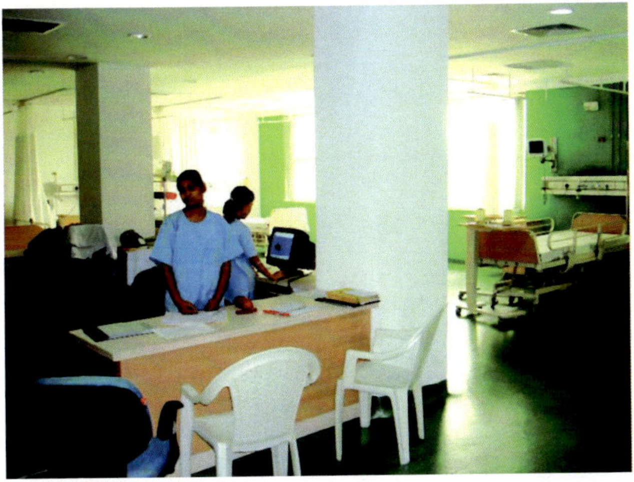

Fig. 4.4: Nursing station plays an important part for patient monitoring

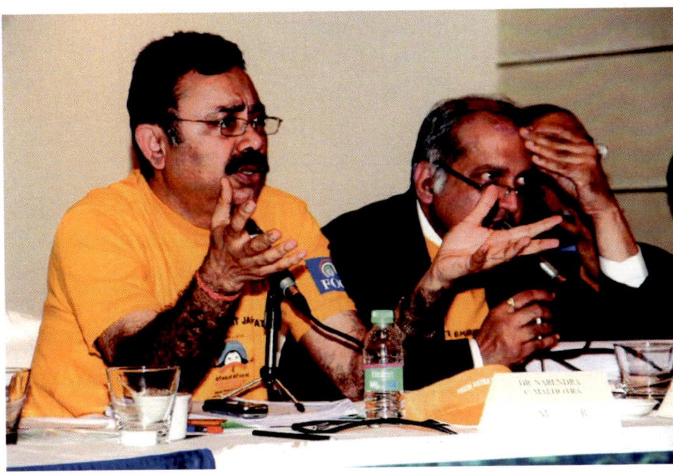

Fig. 4.5: Dr Narendra Malhotra addressing the media as FOGSI President

patient comes through successive zones and finally to OT complex through a hold-up lobby where the trolley change is effected; this area is known as the transfer zones, namely, sterile zones, which include operation theater, anesthesia sterile store theater work, plaster room.

CLEAN ZONE

This includes reception, recovery, instruments store, disposal zone and dirty zone. The soiled instruments and dressings are moved to this area for washing and sterilization. If includes sluice room and dirty wash up, including the sink room and a special corridor serving them. There should be no communication between the first zone and the disposal zone. Ventilation is so organized that air- flows from the sterile zone into the other zones. Thus, a positive air pressure helps to maintain an aseptic area. This has to be carefully implemented by the architect while planning the department.

Ancillary and supporting rooms which have a direct relationship with OT are as follows:

Pre-operational Room

The concept of grouping a number of theaters in one department, so that a number of patients arrive in swift succession, calls for pre-operation room where patients can be prepared for operation. The sitting of this room should be near the "aseptic zone" and connected through a transfer zone.

Recovery Room

The recovery room should be accessible from the hospital site without having to cross the "aseptic zone" and they

Flow chart 4.4: Systems and designs of operation theaters

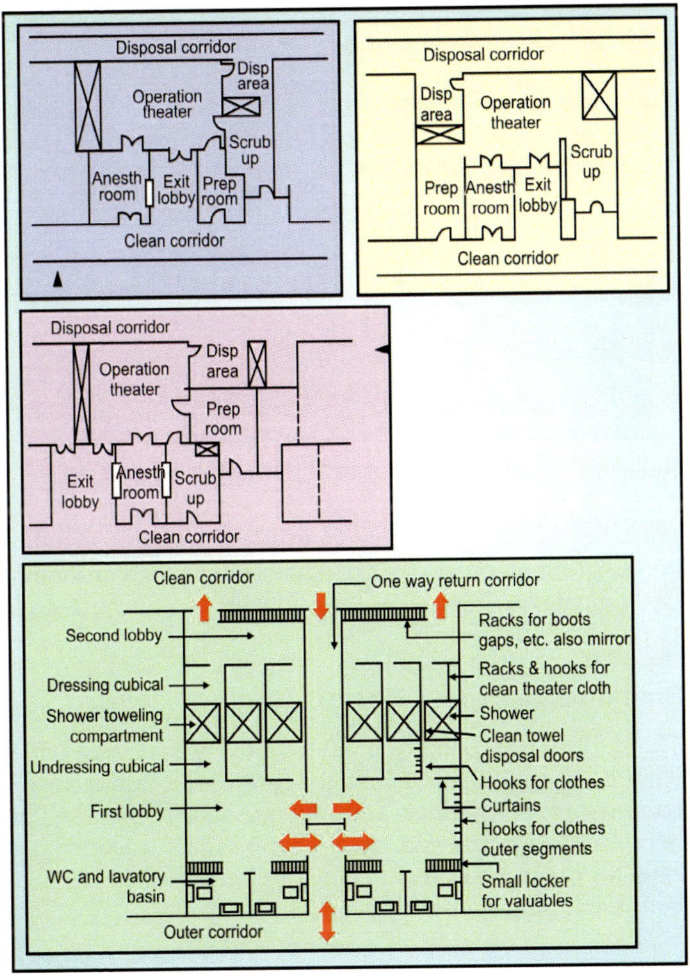

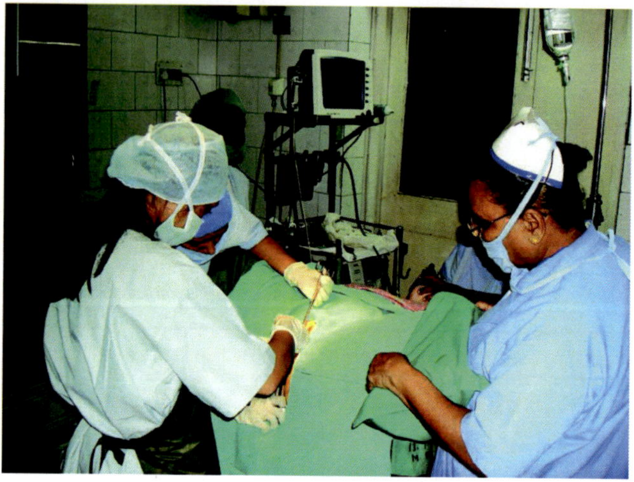

Fig. 4.6: The importance of surgery and its planning thereof

must be directly accessible from OT through a transfer zone. An allowance of one and a half bed per theater should be adequate for the recovery area, depending on the degree of post-anesthetic care.

Staff Change Room

The staff change room should be so sited as to be accessible from both aseptic and clean corridor and a buffer space comprising sets of toilets and shower should be infused in between the air lock and shape change and surgeon and a nursing room, so that they are sterilized and fumigated before entering the sterile corridor.

Plaster Room

This room will be required to perform certain plaster work immediately after operation and it is preferable to site it in

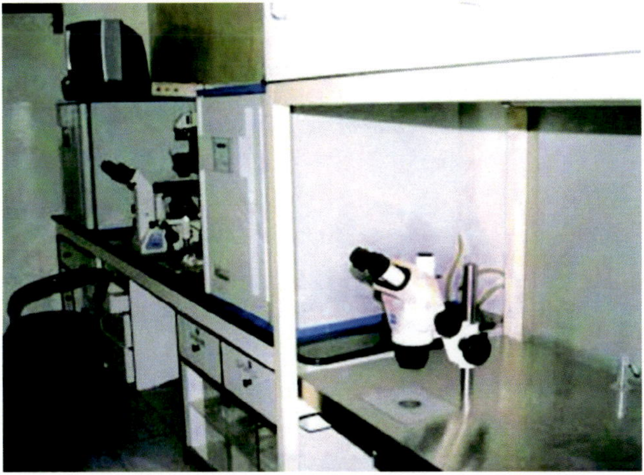

Fig. 4.7: Expensive equipment needs to be protected

the sterile complex. Some experts feel that the plaster room should be outside the OT complex so as to avoid possible infection while making plaster.

CSSD

Due to heavy demand placed by the operating department on the CSSD, their relationship is very vital. It is thus desirable to locate it close to the operation theater.

X-ray Department

X-ray examination of patients is sometimes necessary during or immediately after surgery, as the patients may not be in a position to be taken for X-ray, hence, provision of a mobile X-ray unit should be made.

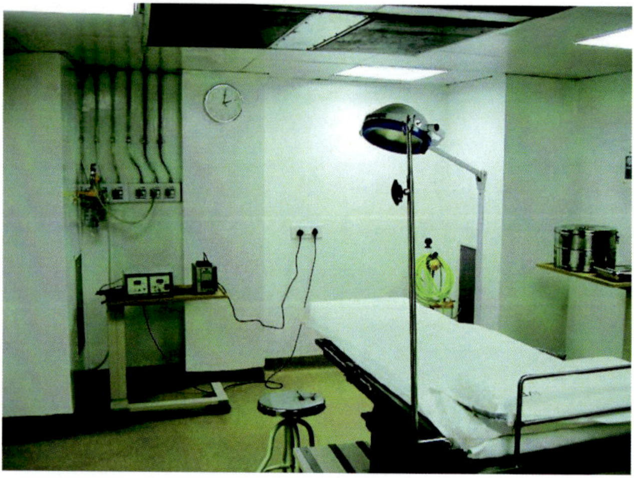

Fig. 4.8: Minor OT

Laboratory

Normally, specimens need to be examined immediately in the OT complex in a small room for post-operation work. Hence, a small lab should be provided.

ICU

It is preferable to site ICU close to the operation theater so as to take advantage of the facilities for outpatients. It should be near the transfer zone and the recovery ward for easy transfer of patient to OT.

Special Fixtures and Fittings

The following special fittings and fixtures are required to be provided in various wards and departments other than operation theater and intensive care unit:

a. Exhaust fan to extract foul air in sanitary annexes, film developing dark room, kitchen and laboratories.
b. Bed pan sink and slab for washing mackintoshes in dirty wash and sluice of normal ward unit with additional item of destructor for special ward unit of infectious disease, pediatric and skin center.
c. Crockery sterilization arrangement in ward kitchen and servey of infectious disease ward and pediatric ward.
d. Large sink for soaking infected linen in infectious disease ward and sink with draining board in all treatment rooms.
e. Central piped fuel gas for ward kitchen, dispensary and laboratories.
f. View windows in sister duty room for constant observation.
g. Steel fabric or concrete jali for psychiatric ward to prevent accidents.
h. Bed side lamp for each patient for reading purposes. These may be fixed on walls.
i. Softened water supply to dispensary and laboratories.
j. Swan neck laboratory type tap for sinks in dispensary and laboratories.
k. Inlet and outlet pipes for fountain spittoons in dental surgery.
l. Plastic trap for wash hand basin and sink in plaster rooms (Dental Center and Operation Theater Department).
m. Acid and alkali proof top for laboratory benches, work benches in clinical test laboratories and loading bench in film developing dark room.
n. Cassette hatches with double compartment exposed and unexposed in wall between radiography and dark room.

o. Non-skid tiles for bottom of hydrotherapy tank.
p. Fume cupboard in specific laboratories.
q. Stainless steel sink and draining board in autopsy room.

Location

In view of the following bacteriological considerations, there is a great need for situating the OT in some kind of cul-de-sac away from the hospital through fare. It should be regarded functionally by the architect as a sterile zone in which traffic other than that specific to the theater must not be permitted.

Hospital Management

Coordination between outdoor, indoor speciality areas, operation theaters and words are of utmost importance. Effective utilization of manpower and material is the culmination of effective management.

CIRCULATION

Normally, there are three types of traffic flow : (i) Patients, (ii) staff, and (iii) supplies. All these three should be properly channelized.

Patients

Patients are brought from the ward and they should not cross the transfer area in their ward clothing, which is a great source of infection. It is in this zone that change-over of the trolley should be effected. The transfer zone will link up the pre-op and recovery areas.

Staff

The surgeon, nurse, sister, nursing orderly should enter through a separate route and through a set of change rooms and through an air lock; they should communicate with the surgical corridor. A shoe change near the air lock is also a necessity.

Supply

All sterile goods should have a different entry point reaching the clean corridor independently. Soiled stuff should get out from the supply only. Non-disposable stuff should go back through the disposable corridor. This way the clean and dirty stuff will not get mixed up, leaving no chance for any infection.

Air Circulation

This should be so arranged that air-flows from the clean to the unclean zones and never vice versa. Otherwise, the clean areas get contaminated.

COMFORT CONDITIONS

Operations sometimes may continue for a long period (4 to 5 hours). This is a nerve cracking job with tremendous mental and physical strain. Hence, optimum comfort level is of vital importance. Some amenities like pantry for refreshments should be made available to the staff. The temperature should be 60 to 70°C with 50 percent humidity. Ventilation must be good with 8 to12 air changes per hour. Staff should also have some room where they can relax. Occasionally, the surgeon may like to dictate postoperation notes in his room.

SAFETY CONSIDERATIONS

With the increased use of volatile anesthetics, the risk of explosion is high and proper precautions need to be taken.

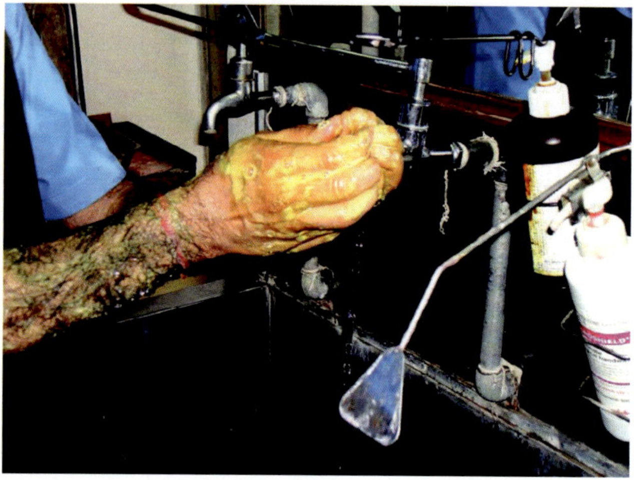

Fig. 4.9: Safe planning of washing area

The possible sources are as follows:

a. Direct contact: Open flame from gas, sterilizers.
b. Faulty loose electrical connection and apparatus.
c. Static electricity which is produced due to friction with the floor either with shoes or wheels or moving equipment.

For (a) and (b) above, adequate firefighting is a must as well as periodic checking of all connections and equipment. For (c) a special antistatic flooring, which carries away the electricity, should be provided in all areas were volatile anesthetic gases are used.

OTHER ENGINEERING SERVICES

Ventilation, air conditioning, heating, hot and cold water, piped suction oxygen and medical gases and electricity are the major services which are to be provided. With ever-changing technology and developing medical science, lot of new gadgets are coming into use and hence the electricity layout should be flexible enough to take care of new developments. Concealed conduit wiring should be provided as a means of fire protection. Provision of two way intercom and closed circuit TV for educational purposes is needed, particularly for teaching establishments. It is desirable to put socket outlets around be avoided. A height of 18 inches above the floor avoids the damage caused by water. A very important aspect in vertical communication is an efficient lift service in multistorey hospitals. As a stand by, ramp connecting various floors is provided.

Provision of stand-by generating sets and alternative sources of power supply must be planned so that, in case of breakdown, the supply gets restored automatically. The

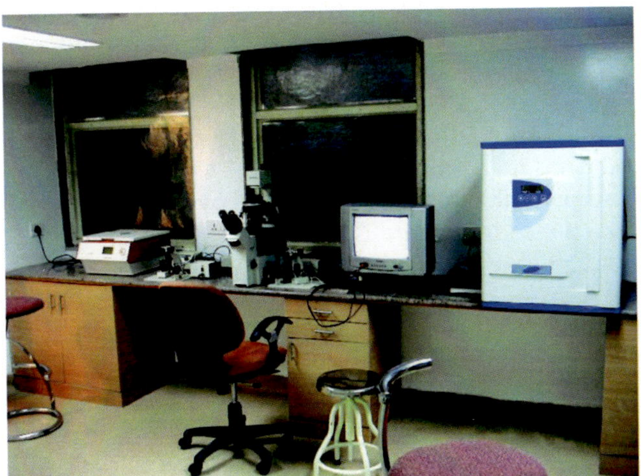

Fig. 4.10: Safety of the equipment and people working

other method is "NO BREAK SUPPLY". One of the lifts feeding the OT block must be fed by this alternative supply.

Lighting of OT

This needs to be carefully planned, as most of the operations are performed under artificial light. From lighting considerations, OT has three distinct functional areas, each having specific requirements.

i. The surgeons field.
ii. The anesthetics field.
iii. The general lighting.

Surgeon's Field

This is the important operational area where lighting should reach near perfection. The problem is that the actual operation is often at the bottom of a cavity with a slant axis 6 to 12, inches deep. The heads of the surgeon and his assistants continuously intervene in the light source and the objects. The operation field also changes as the operation proceeds. Hence, there is need to have a highly, flexible illumination system capable of being redirected easily and instantly.

At present, the job is done with an overhead shadowless lamp, but indeed there is scope for research in this field. In fact, the overhead light, unless housed properly, may collect dust, which is liable to fall on the affected areas or instruments when tilted. Thus, it is imperative to house the, electrical fittings properly.

Anesthetics Field

The anesthetist gets important indications of the patient's condition, by visual examination of his face, eyes and lips, etc. Here, lighting must be approximate to daylight. Too much red may give rise to glare and unduly favorable conditions, while too much blue will create the reverse impression. Besides the anesthetist will have to read and keep track of monitoring instruments and this makes good daylight conditions, imperative.

General Lighting

This must be such that the theater sister and staff can select and manipulate instruments with care, viz threading of the needles with fine sutures. There is an advantage in having large elements of daylighting; these create pleasant working conditions for the staff who might feel trapped without any windows to the world outside. Of course arrangements for darkening should also be made.

SPECIFICATIONS

Windows

These should be dust-proof with rubber gaskets and double glazing for air conditioning purposes. The opening should be upto 15 percent of floor area.

Doors

The doors should be wide enough for easy movement of stretchers and trolleys. These could be of double action and two-leaf type with 5 feet widths.

Floors

There should be *in situ* mosaic floors with least possible joints with brass/copper stripes 6 inches apart both ways to carry away any static electricity produced by earthing. These should be provided wherever risk of anesthetic gas explosion is there, viz, OT/ICU recovery, pre-operative rooms, anesthesia rooms, etc.

Walls

In situ mosaic finish for full height of walls, is necessary.

Ceiling

The ceiling must have cement plaster with washable paint. Corners of all operations theater rooms should be rounded off to prevent collection of dirt and dust.

Scrub-up

Sinks should be knee operated. A viewing panel should be provided for the surgeon to observe the OT activities while scrubbing his hands.

Electrical Wiring

It should be of concealed type and there should be no projection inside the OT wall surface. All fittings should be flush with wall surfaces.

Power Points

Power points for spot lights, diathermy apparatus, electric saw and similar electric appliances should be planned.

INTENSIVE CARE UNIT PREAMBLE

In this unit, critically ill patients requiring highly skilled life-saving medical aid and nursing care round the clock are concentrated. These include major surgical and medical cases, and patients with head injuries, severe hemorrhages, kidney and respiratory catastrophic poisoning and so on.

In short, the ultimate medicare hospital must be equipped with highly specialized staff and equipment.

By segregating the critically ill patients who really need the above mentioned care/treatment, the general wards can be separately provided for. Care should however, be taken that only critically ill patients are admitted to this unit, otherwise, the whole purpose of specialized treatment will be defected. As soon as the patient recovered from the critical stage, he or she must be removed to general ward nursing unit to avoid unnecessary overcrowding.

LOCATION

This unit should be sited close to the operation theater and near to the other essential departments, X-ray and pathology laboratory, so that the staff and ancillaries could be shared. Easy and convenient access from emergency casualty department is also essential. Besides, this unit will also need all the specialized service such as suction medical gases, no-break electric supply, heating, ventilation, air conditioning and efficient lift services as are needed for an operation theater. A good natural light and pleasant environment will be of great help psychologically for the patients and staff, so that they may not feel that they are cut off from the rest of the world.

SIZE

In armed forces hospitals, the intensive care unit caters for 26 percent of authorized bed strength of the hospitals. The unit should be as small as feasible but no more than 6.8 beds in a group. A larger unit will tend to be noisy, because practically all patients in this unit will need frequent assistance. Intensive care is meant to give a critically ill patient the best medical care to survive. It is very important to see that the staff entrusted to keep watch and help them in nursing their trouble are not over-fatigued and they can maintain their composure and balance in moments of stress/crisis.

FLOOR SPACE

The floor space per bed in this unit should be higher than the general bed space to cater for free movement, check against cross infection and at times utilization of specialized bulky equipment. The scales provide 140 FS per bed for the unit. It should be possible to screen off each bed. It will be advantageous to plan a couple of beds in isolated glazed cubicles for cases which need complete segregation for various reasons.

BASIC PLANNING

The basic consideration in planning should be to have (i) a fully visible patient area with adequate space all around for positioning life-saving equipment, (ii) a central nurse station with minimum possible walking distance for the nurses/sister, (iii) an adequate stock of medicines, emergency packs and the like, and (iv) distinct clean and dirty utility areas where movement of staff and supplies could be controlled.

Patients' Area

Natural light is desirable and should be provided as far as possible, but glare and direct sunrays falling on the patients bed must be avoided. The positions of fittings and fixtures is very important, as each patient may require the use of several items of equipment which have to be connected to outlets. Screen for curtaining off patients should be of light and cleanable material and easy to handle too.

Nurses Station

This should be planned as on open area with adequate counter- space for writing, telephones, patients monitoring equipment, X-ray, viewing boxes, etc. Open planning is adopted for visibility as well as audibility of the entire patient area. A small pantry space along the nurses station is helpful.

Clean Utility Area

This should contain all the essential supplies, linen, medicines, lotions, syringes, trolleys for various mobile equipment needs, medical gases, sterilizers, constant water supply with appropriate sinks, preferably elbow or knee operated.

Clinical Room

This should cater to the need of immediate clinical tests and investigations. All essential testing devices must be properly housed in it.

Artificial Lighting

The patient's area should be uniformly lit free from glare of any sort. All such fittings should have control from centrally placed nurses duty station. Adjustment to dim light should be possible. In case high intensity light is required, provisions to supplement general lighting with portable lamps should be available. Lighting beneath the beds will also be needed to check drainage of bottles and under-bed seals. Nurses station should have adequate working light intensity, but should not be a source of disturbance to the patient. A good direct light over work benches in the clean utility area should be provided.

Chapter 5

Medical Clinics

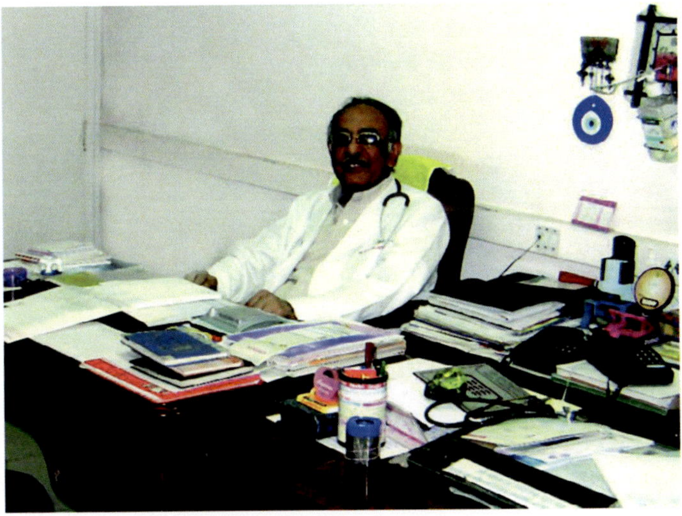

A senior Dr RM Malhotra in his clinic.

CLINICS

The word clinic comes from the Greek word "Klinikos" meaning bed ridden patients. As time passed, the word became more literal. It became an institution or station for outpatients, so clinic is for consultation without in-house facilities and it is special for every field. Which can be divided into:

1. Medicine Gen.
2. Surgery
3. Gynecology and obstetrics
4. Antenatal
5. Pediatrics.
6. Orthopedics
7. Skin and dermatology
8. Ophthalmology: eye
9. ENT
10. Dental
11. Heart Clinic
12. Psychiatric
13. X-ray and Diagnostic
14. IVF clinics
15. Physiotherapy
16. Nursing homes
17. Large hospitals
18. Ayurvedic/skin clubs/slimming centers/special clinics.

Special Therapies

- Sujok
- Reiki
- Ayurveda/massages
- Slimming clubs/diet clinic

Flow chart 5.1: Arrangement of various activity rooms in a system

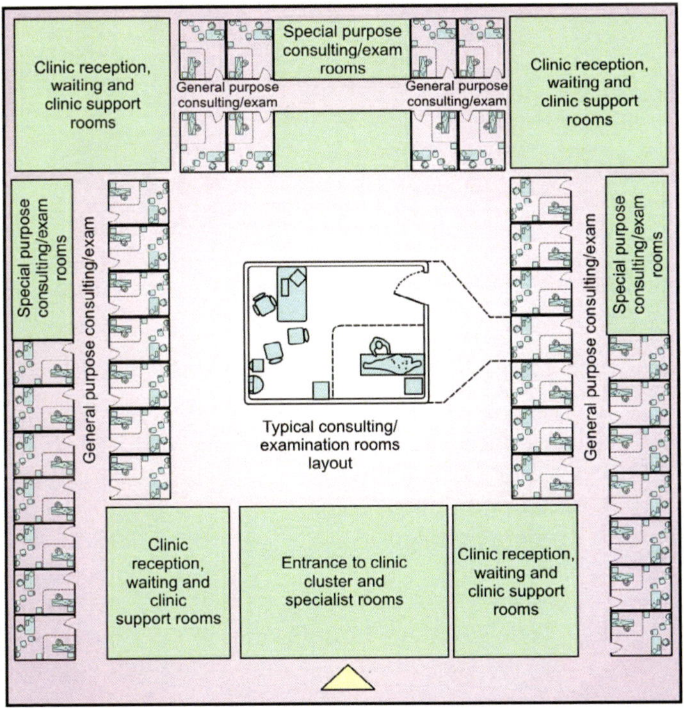

- Health clubs/spa/gym
- Special clubs for disabled children with learning disability
- Awareness clinics for children and sex education
- Sex education
- AIDS awareness
- Drug de-addiction
- Homeopathic clinic
- Counselling clinics.

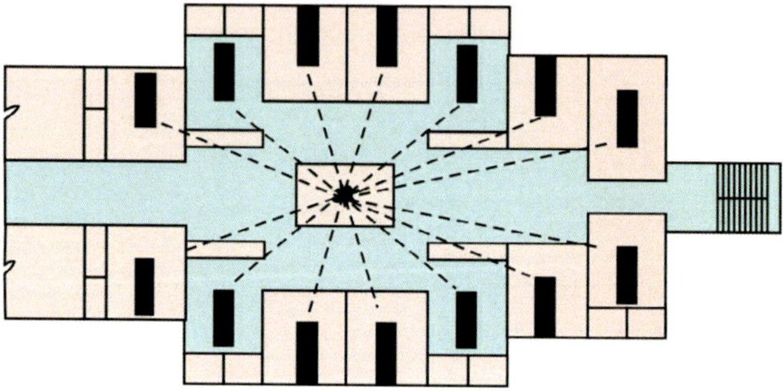

Fig. 5.1: Combining some advantages of circular and rectangular units

MINIMUM OFFICE AREAS [CLINIC]

1. Waiting room = 10 × 12 = 120 sq. ft.
2. Receptionist = 6 × 10 = 60 sq. ft.
3. Doctor's consultation = 10 × 10 = 100 sq. ft.
4. Two examining rooms = 2 × 8 × 10 = 160 sq. ft.
5. General storage = 3 × 5 = 15 sq. ft.
6. Laboratory = 8 × 10 = 80 sq. ft.
7. X-ray = 9 × 10 = 90 sq. ft.
8. 2 Toilets (1 staff, 1 public) = 2 × 5 × 6 = 60 sq. ft.

X-RAY

1. X-ray room = 12 × 15 = 180 sq. ft.
2. Dark room = 6 × 8 = 48 sq. ft.
3. Storage room control = 8 × 15 = 120 sq. ft.
4. 2 Dressing alcoves = 2 × 4 × 6 = 48 sq. ft.

SURGERY

1. Surgery scrub up sink = 10 × 13 = 130 sq. ft.
2. One cast and injection room = 10 × 13 = 130 sq. ft.
3. One central supply of services = 8 × 15 = 120 sq. ft.

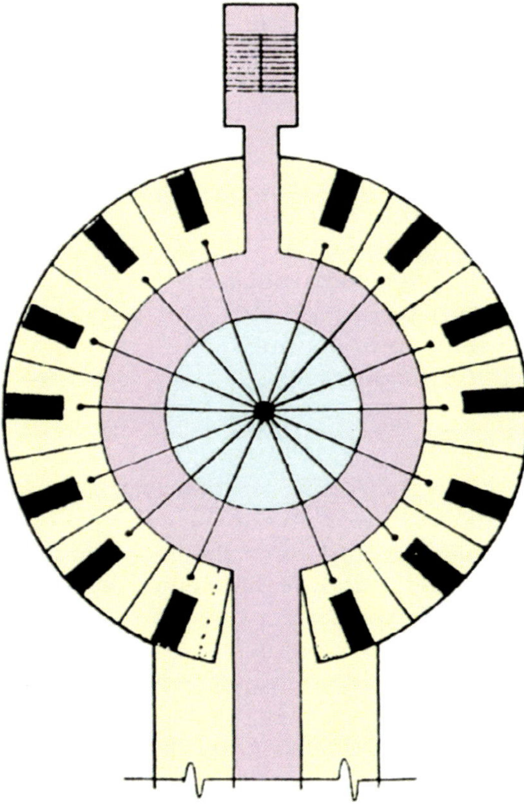

Fig. 5.2: Circular pattern with all patients equidistant from the nurse

General Observations of a Clinic

1. Information systems.
2. Clarity in sign posts.
3. Adequate information in communication language.
4. In-built fear of patient should be taken.

5. Need for privacy.
6. Personal inhibition.
7. Security.
8. Cleanliness.
9. Accountability.
10. Manageability.
11. Circulation.
12. Sequence of space.
13. Materials.
14. Lighting and ventilator.
15. Services.
16. Built-in equipment.
17. Air conditioning.

GENERAL MEDICINE

- General medicine practitioners can be put in a single room space or have an organized space.
- For a solo practitioner, the amount of space needed will depend entirely on his method of practice.
- Waiting room = 6′ × 12′ = 120 sq. ft.
- Receptionist = 60 sq. ft.
  (Combination of nurse and bookkeeper)
- Consultant office 10′ × 10′= 100 sq. ft.
- Examination cabin (two = 80 sq. ft. each)

SURGERY

General Requirements

- Reception
- Waiting
- Consultation
- Examination
- Minor OT

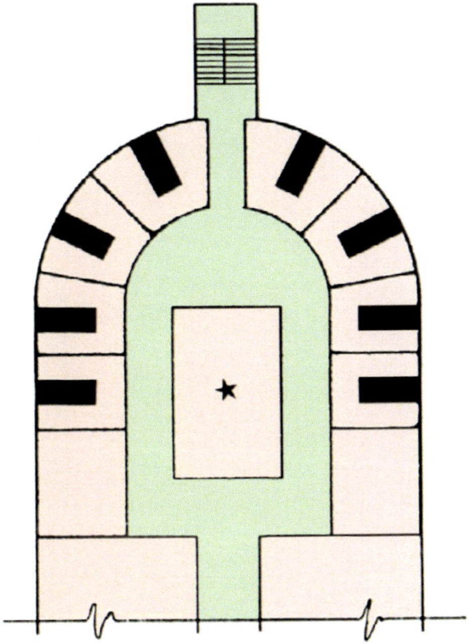

Fig. 5.3: Patients in a semicircle with utilities in remainder of area

- Recovery Room
- Nurse Room
- Toilet

Technical Requirements

- Surgeon reception counter and waiting hall
- Doctor's consultancy chamber and examination room (3′-10″ wide door)
- Dressing room
- Minor procedure room for septic and non-septic cases.

Flowchart 5.2: Typical intensive therapy unit layout

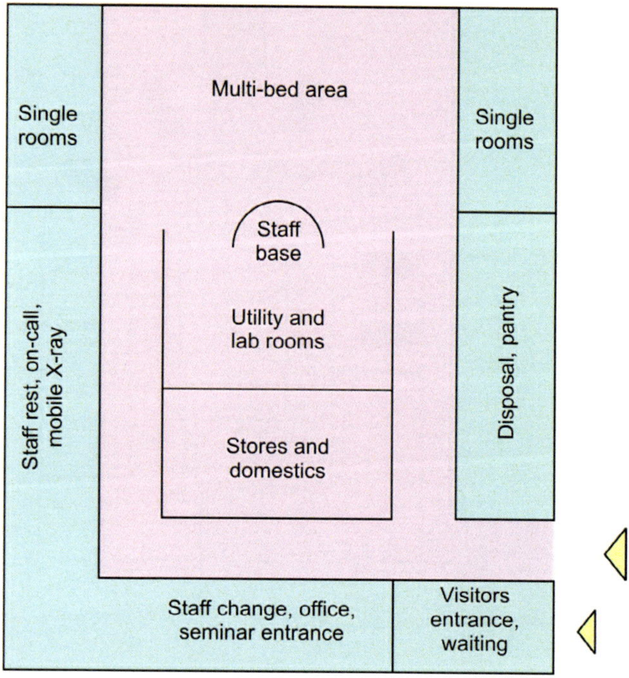

- Bathroom for doctor's and nurses with special provision for washing used linen.
- Separate changing room for OT staff.
- Changing room for doctors, equipped with racks for clothes, lockers for personal belongings, masks and caps, racks for slippers to be provided.
- Scrub room (for nurses and doctors) equipped with washbasins, with elbow action water taps, geysers.
- Sterilization room equipped with sterilizers, OTI care

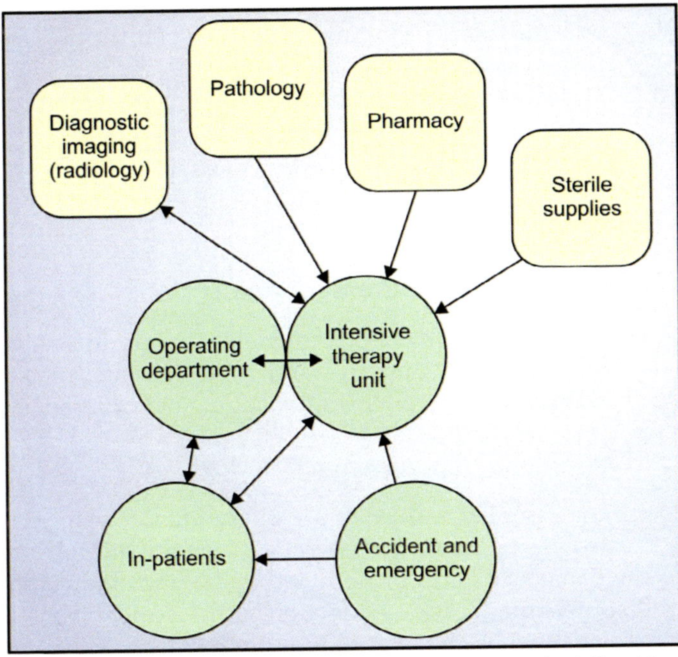

Fig. 5.4: Intensive therapy unit (ITU): Interdepartmental relationship

for formalization, cooking gas, storage facilities for sterilized drums

- Operation theater.

AC room equipped with hydraulic OT table, OT light ceiling, Boyle's apparatus, pulse oximeter, suction motor.

It must be equipped with an exhaust fan and facility to seal the room during formalization of the room.

(Walls should be of ceramic tiles to facilitate washing and cleaning).

- Recovery room attached with bathroom and life-saving

equipment including central oxygen supply, monitor and suction motor.

- Private room with attached toilet/bath, with facility of attendant's bed (min. 5).
- Generator room with investor central supply oxygen.
- Staff room
- Staff kitchenette and toilet.

Sterilization and Storage Area

It is not possible to perform major surgery in small clinic, so only minor surgeries and post-operative results and examination are done and changing of bordered, etc.

Operating Department

The essential feature of an 'operating department' is the provision of a 'sterile' operating room for the performance of major surgical procedures, so that they may be carried out without risk of infection to the patient. This end is achieved by the operating room being positively pressurised in relation to the surrounding rooms, and the air supply to it being passed through filters. In standard theaters an air change rate of 20 changes per hour is effective. However, a number of surgical procedures require a higher standard of sterility. These are procedures where any degree of infection would result in the operation being unsuccessful. Typical of this group is hip replacement surgery, but the 'ultra clean' conditions are also called for in any joint replacement procedure or when any 'foreign' implant is being introduced into the body (e.g. stents).

Provisions of 'ultra clean' conditions is achieved by the use of so-called 'sterile enclosures' within which a vertical laminar flow of high volumes of filtered air is achieved. It should be noted that while laminar flow has been shown to be very successful in minimizing infection rates in joint replacement surgery, it has shown no such benefits in the broader range of general surgery. In view of the large volumes of air that need to be pumped through enclosures to ensure an effective laminar flow pattern, this is also a costly ventilation option.

The remaining areas of the operating theater suite, in addition to the operating room itself, may be categorized into three zones:

- An inner 'high sterility' zone where conditions akin to those in the operating room are required, and which contains the preparation room where instrument trolleys are laid up, the anesthetic room, and the scrub-up and gowning room.
- An outer zone, still within the protected confines of the theater suite, consisting of staff changing rooms, showers, toilets, staff rest rooms where breaks during operating lists may be taken.
- The entry zone which may also contain offices, stores and laboratories.

The entire operating theaters suite must be tightly controlled at the entry point, at which transfer of the patient from bed or trolley should take place to prevent contamination of the theater environment.

Day Surgery

Already 70 percent of elective surgery is in many places being carried out on a day basis, and this proportion is still increasing. Day surgery units are often provided as completely free-standing units but for safety's sake, as well as for the ability to share back-up services, there is a case for them being located in a hospital.

Where all surgical services are centralized at the DGH,

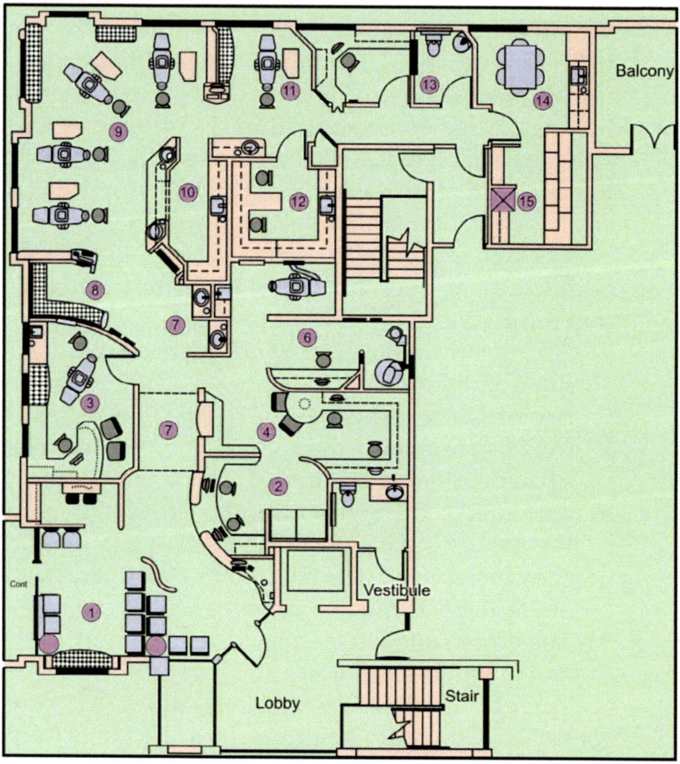

Fig. 5.5: Floor plan 2

there is dilemma as to whether the main operating theaters should cater for day surgical patients or whether a separate day surgical unit (DSU) should be provided. The latter may be conveniently located near a hospital entrance and car park. However, as day surgery patients this location should be balanced against the possibly stronger needs of other departments to be readily accessible from car parks.

From a utilization point of view, there is an advantage

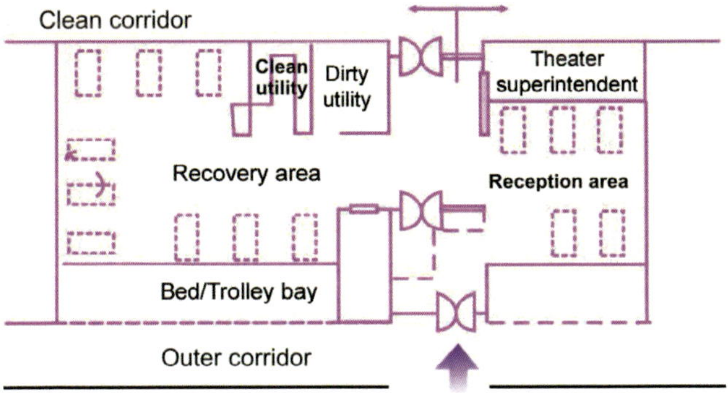

Fig. 5.6: Placement of recovery area

in the use of main theaters for day surgery: as day surgery will generally decline. There are also economies in staffing, supplies and other back-up services, and in air-conditioning and other engineering plant. Where the main theaters are used for day surgery there must be separate day surgery facilities-reception, consulting, pre-operative waiting and post-operative recovery—which should be easily accessible from an external entrance.

If larger acute hospitals are linked to and supported by locality hospitals, as outlined in the 'Future strategies' example, then day surgery would generally take place in units at the locality hospitals.

One or more endoscopy rooms will generally be provided as part of the day surgical unit. They may have their own recovery area. The operating theaters need to be designed to the same size and standards as those provided for in-patients. In some DSUs anesthetic rooms are omitted, and anesthetic is administered in the theater.

It is important to know whether patients will go to a bed area, change and leave their clothes there, and return there after surgery, or whether they will go straight from a changing room to the theater suite. In the latter case their belongings will be taken to the bed area where they will recover.

GYNE

- Reception and counter
- Waiting room
- Record room
- Staff room
- Linen room sheets, gowns, masks, etc. and needles, syringes, scissors, etc. are stored
- Attendant's kitchenette
- Washing area
- Sterilization room. All the instruments are sterilized against infection
- Baby vaccination room. He/she is made active and attended
- Labor room. Normal delivery active and attended.
- Major operation theater surgery is carried out
- Minor operation theater
- Private rooms with attached bathroom.

Note: Private rooms and OT should be for apart.

Zoning/Grouping

- Labor room, vaccination room, operation theater, sterilization room, washing area, emergency room
- Private rooms with attached toilets
- Staff room, attendant's kitchenette, washing room, linen room, stationary room, record room
- Reception, counter, waiting room, toilet.

Maternity

- 75 beds cater for 2700 delivers/year
- 100 beds cater for 3600
- 125 beds cater for 4500.

Maternity Clinic

- Antenatal
- Postnatal
- Baby following
- Family planning.

Backup

- Reception
- Administration
- Records
- Provision for education.

Delivery Suit

- Theater
- Abnormal and normal delivery room
- Assessment area.

Obstetric Theater Suit

- Theater (28 m^2) with full mechanical ventilator
- Humidity and cooling control
- Antistatic flooring
- Oxygen and nitrous oxide
- Two vacuum points for mother
- Vacuum and oxygen for baby
- Scrub for growing areas (9.5 m^2)
- Anesthetic room (16.5 m^2)

- Recovery beds for 2 patients (25 m^2)
- Clean utility (8.5 m^2).

  Delivery room require pleasant day light environment with privacy (blinds to windows) good lighting for suturing sound attenuation, anti-static precautions, medical gas, oxygen and vacuum outlets, and mechanical ventilation with humidity and cooling installations.
- Abnormal delivery room (24 m^2 + scrub area 1.5 m^2).
- Normal delivery room (15 m^2).

Area Assessment

- Twenty percent beds should be in 1-bed wards (13 m^2/bed) with oxygen outlet at bed head.
- Eighty percent beds should be in multi-bed bays (9.5 m^2/bed) with oxygen outlet to each pair of beds.

Special Care Baby Unit (SCBU)

- Multi-cot bays (4 m^2/cot)
- Single-cot room (5.5 m^2)
- Special-cot room (7.5 m^2).

Must include

- Gowning and hand wash areas for visitors
- Changing accommodation for staff
  - Female (11-14 m^2)
  - Male (7.5 m^2)
- Bed sitting room per mothers with shower and wc
- First stage of labor—Obstetrics
- Room should be private, available to the husband and furnished as in a home
- Facilities of radio, TV plus washroom and toilet facilities should be there

- The lounge should allow room for the woman to walk as it aids easy birth.
- In the labor, delivery room, attention should be given to comforts and facilities.
- Organisation of ancillary services must be provided for constant supervision and two way communication.
- The services of the obstetric suite should relate to care of patient, not to processing of supplies. The central service department, linen and folding service and central dispatch area should have control over the supply function.

Maternity

Childbirth is a natural process, but one that may occasionally threatens the life or health of both mother and child, and this presents dilemmas for designers of maternity units. For the great majority of cases, a stay of only a day or two is enough. Traditionally the components of a maternity unit are the antenatal clinic, wards (mainly post-natal, but also for the few who need observation before birth), the delivery suite, and the neonatal (or special care baby) unit. With ever shortening lengths of stay, the logic of separation of delivery suite and post-natal ward has been questioned. The alternative, pioneered in UK at Kingston Hospital, is the LDRP (labor, delivery, recovery, post-partum) room. This room is fully equipped as a normal delivery room, but with domestic décor and equipment located out of sight, and toilet and small sluice en suite- is accepted by the mother for the whole of her stay. An abnormal delivery room and full operating theater are still needed for cesarean and other more difficult births. There is also likely to be demand for one or more water-birthing rooms. The LDPR arrangement has the

Flow chart 5.3: Typical small hospital

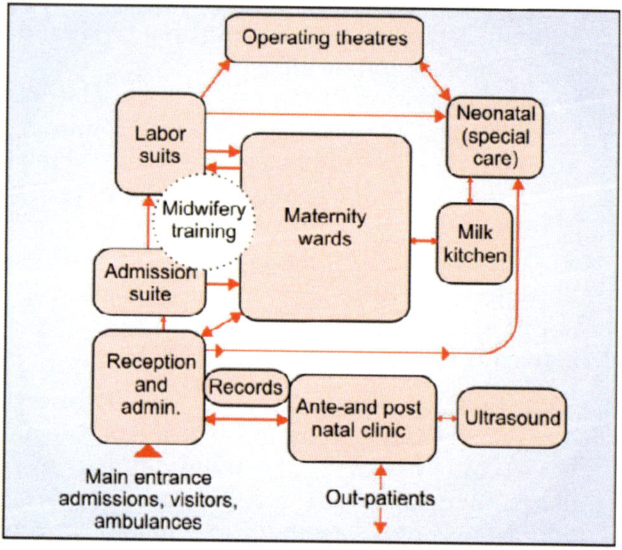

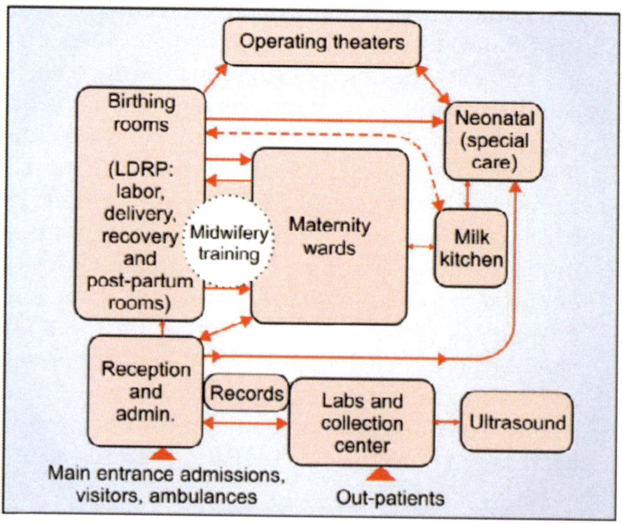

disadvantage of a lack of the company of other mothers, which is more important for some than for others, so a day room is needed. Waiting facilities for the expectant fathers pose an acute problem that arises in many parts of the hospital: here, above all, the dangers of smoking need emphasis, but this is a stressful situation and one particularly difficult for smokers. Groups of smokers are often seen huddled outside entrances to many hospitals. A possible solution is a small well-ventilated room with a separately ventilated lobby between it and any other corridor. This lobby might be approached directly from the draught lobby at hospital entrances.

The antenatal clinic in a large hospital will be fully utilized throughout the week, and may usefully be sometimes open outside normal hours. The traditional design with three-sided examining rooms open to a shared corridor is no longer acceptable: convenient for doctors, it denies to the expectant mother the necessary privacy for confidential talk. A combined consulting/examining room, such as is found in OPDs, is the preferred solution. In smaller hospitals, the antenatal clinic could take place in the general OPD, provided that the waiting and other ancillary spaces are for exclusive maternity use during these clinics.

A neonatal unit is needed for any major maternity department. There is controversy about the required size—many have been built larger than has ever been needed. Very high levels of engineering services, particularly of socket outlets and temperature control, are required. Many babies will be in incubators, some (where isolation is needed) in single rooms. Every facility must be given to maximize parent's contact with their babies. Some longer stay babies, and those needing surgery, will have to be transferred to more specialized units.

In a hospital with a patient-focused emphasis, the maternity unit may form part of a 'women and children's hospital'. In any case, it is an advantage for the children's wards and services in the hospital to be near the maternity unit, for ease of access by pediatricians. The obstetricians are usually also responsible for gynecology wards and outpatients.

PEDIATRIC

- Clinic should be acceptable to child psyche.
- Reception
- Waiting
- Consultation chamber should be such that children are not scared.
- Instead of an examination table, doctor to examine a child can use a soft bed.
- Place for vaccination
- Place for nebulisers
- Proper light, ventilation-bright interiors
- Concealed medicine storage
- No unpleasant smells in the clinic
- Weight scale, growth chart, height measurement
- Colorful interiors, toys, etc.
- Colorful informative health charts.

ORTHOPEDICS

- Reception
- Waiting
- X-ray for immediate treatment
- Plaster room
- OT for surgery
- Recovery room
- Records/administrative.

EYE SPECIALIST

- Reception/counter and waiting hall
- Toilet for staff
- Staff room
- Doctor's room. Well-equipped with slit-lamp, keratometer, A scan, B scan.
- Optometrist room will be equipped with auto-reflectometer, trial set, slit-lamp, retinascope and contact lens trial set.
- Laser room equipped with lasik laser, green laser, yag laser.
- Perimetry Room field test is done.
- Operation theater.
  - — Autoclaving room
  - — Changing room
  - — Main OT.
- Wards with attached toilet
- Optical section
- Angiography room (photographs of retina are taken).
- Record room, accounts room
- Chemist shop/Pharmacy
- Kitchenette.

DENTAL CLINIC

Dental clinic is a bit different from normal clinic.

- Requires reception, waiting, information, consultation room and works room in itself.
- Dental chair which takes space of 4′× 6′ is the main equipment for dentist.
- For small dental clinic around 200 sq. ft. area is enough.
- Chairs can be placed side by side or in radical pattern.
- X-ray is an integral part, which is near a chair or in bigger clinic. There can be a small room which taken full mouth X-ray 8′ × 6′ is enough.

- Workstation is required near all chairs.
- Small lab required, area 100 sq. ft.
- Developer X-ray area
- Photography area
- Model making area
- Toilets
- Counseling room.

X-ray and Diagnostic Center

- Waiting room
- Reception and counter : 15′ × 11′-2″
- X-ray room : (13′-8″× 18′)
- Ultrasound room : (18′ × 13′- 8″)
- ECG room
- Fully computerised lab
- Sterilization room
- Analysis room/dark room (13′ × 9′-8″)
- Record room and storage room. Records of patients are kept
- Staff room
- Staff's kitchenette (4′ × 5′)
- Toilets
- Small changing room
- Reporting room
- Film collection room (15′ × 8′).

Diagnostic Center

- Reception/Counter (15′ × 11′- 2″)
- Waiting hall
- Toilet
- Sample collection room
- Doctor's room

- Laboratory
- Microbiology room with attached toilet. Sensitivity test, urine related test, bacteria, fungus.

Diagnostic Imaging

This term embraces diagnostic investigations using X-rays (either as plain films, or making use of contrast media) and the non-X-ray modalities using ultrasound and magnetic resonance to produce images.

The essential feature about planning 'imaging departments' is that, apart from ultrasound, imaging modalities require specialized protective arrangements, either from radiation or from magnetic fields.

Protection in X-ray rooms may be provided by lead or barium plaster which prevent the emission of radiation beyond the room. Where control positions are within the room, lead screens may protect operators. During investigations, staff who must work in close proximity to the patient, may additionally wear lead aprons, and patients themselves may require specific shielding from radiation to sensitive zones such as gonads.

Patients on entry to the imaging department need tranquil reception and waiting areas before moving to the diagnostic rooms. The layout of the department should ensure that frequently used rooms and those whose investigations are brief (e.g. plain X-ray, chest rooms) are sited closest to the waiting areas. All rooms will require patient changing facilities, with fast-throughout rooms requiring a higher proportion than those servicing longer procedure rooms. Changing rooms may be either 'stand-alone' or 'pass-through'. In this later category, the patient accesses the room from the sub-waiting space, and enters the diagnostic room directly from the changing room.

These rooms have the advantage that, once undressed, the patient does not have to traverse any general circulation and so benefits from greater privacy. However, this pattern is often found to be very claustrophobic for patients, and can generate anxieties that one has been placed in this isolated space and forgotten. It is also a pattern, which, because of the more numerous doorways into the X-ray rooms, creates additional problems in achieving radiation protection. The greater flexibility of the stand-alone pattern usually makes it the preferred option.

X-ray rooms, which make use of contrast media, need some facility for preparation. With the simple applications, such as computerised tomography or intravenous pyelogram, a simple utility/preparation is needed, for barium studies, a barium kitchen where the medium can be made up is needed; and for barium enema studies a WC en-suite with the radiography room is vital.

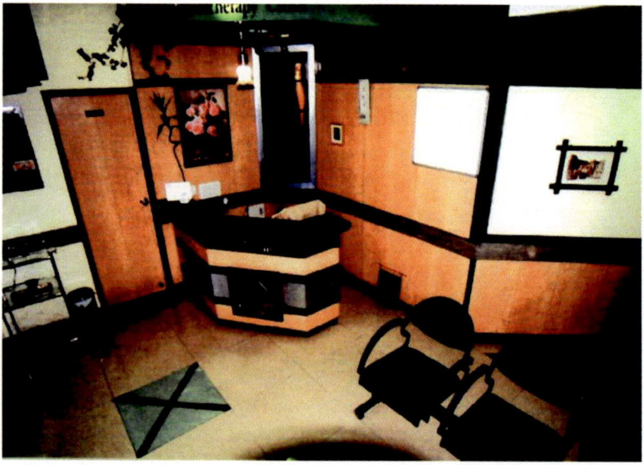

Fig. 5.7: A composed waiting and reception area

Protection from magnetic fields in magnetic resonance imaging studies initially depended on the provision of sufficient area around the magnet for the strength of the field to fall off. However, current trends are for the use of lower testa magnets and for protection from the magnetic field to be built into the machine.

In radiology departments, considerations of radiation protection demand that the diagnostic rooms are internal. In those circumstances it becomes particularly important that the more general spaces, offices, sorting and reporting rooms, and staff rest rooms have natural light.

Most X-ray processing now makes use of daylight processing, and processors can be sited within the staff areas or within general circulation space, which can help to simplify circulation and to create a more compact staff working area. However, some specialist investigations may make use of cine film, and for these a small dark room needs to be provided.

PHYSIOTHERAPY CLINIC

- *Equipment's required:* Neuro-developmental equipment; gait-trainer, walker for cerebral problems.
- Short-wave diathermy, electrical stimulator, ultrasound apparatus, cervical or lumbar traction table, aerodyne, microwave units, wax bath, cold and hot pack units, infrared and ultraviolet lamps, quadriceps table, whirlpools for hydrotherapy.

PHYSIOTHERAPY

- The effectiveness depends on space, location and work areas. Ventilation, lighting, interior finish.
- Occupational and physical therapy should be in close proximity.

- Space required depends on treatments required. Equipment like whirlpool, bath, treatment tables, parallel bars, etc. are minimum essentials for even in a one therapist department.
- Reception area should have adequate space for stretcher and wheel chair patients.
- *Staff space:* Private-office space suitable for interviewing patients, administrative and clerical duties, holding files, writing facilities for dictation, space for staff lockers, dressing rooms separate from the patient area.
- *Examining room:* Floor to ceiling partitions for privacy.
- *Treatment area:*
  1. Cubicle (dry) large enough for therapist to work on either side of the table. Curtains for convenient access divide it with open panels at the top for ventilation when drawn. Lockers are required for outpatients.
  2. Underwater exercise area (wet) including a treatment table with a tank of exercise pool.
  3. Exercise area (open):Flexible open space, used extensively by people in wheel chairs, on crutches/ canes. At least one wall should be reinforced for installation of stall bars.
- *Toilet facilities:* Separate facilities for patients and staff. Patient's facilities to accommodate wheel chair patients, for children, seat adapters with footrest.
- *Storage:* For stretchers, wheel chairs, it is best to plan carport spaces. Simple accessible and well lighted storage.

SPECIAL CONSIDERATIONS

- *Ventilation:* Adequate, controlled ventilation. A continuous, reliable flow of fresh air is essential. Air conditioning is a necessity for some areas in a physiotherapy clinic.

- *Sinks:* Hospital hand washing laboratories with hot and cold water mixing outlets, preferably foot operated at convenient height.
- *Interior finishes:* Activity of patients on wheelchairs/ stretchers subject to heavy wear on floors and walls, remaining attractive yet stand up to the rough usage. *Examples:* Ceramic wall tiles or glazed structural units for walls and floors. Colors that work are 'cool pastels' -green, blue, violet.
- *Doors:* Within the department should be at least 40″ wide. No raised thresholds.
- *Ceiling Moorings:* It is useful for attaching overhead equipment as hoists, pulleys, bars, counter balancing equipment, each supporting at least 500 pounds.

IVF Center

- Waiting reception
- Doctors room + examination chamber
- Counseling room (privacy is most needed)
- Ultrasound room
- MOT
- Sterilization area
- OT
- Lab
- Storage area
- Day ward area + private room

This is very Hi-Tech branch of medical services and total privacy is needed here. Area for small IVF center is around 900 sq. ft. This area should be clean, and sterilized area with lots of privacy. Clean floor, dust free A/c environment is needed.

NURSING HOME

A. Needed by : Patients who do not need permanent hospital care and yet cannot be catered for in residential care homes.

B. Design and accommodation.

In all cases the design of nursing homes should aim at providing as relaxed a domestic atmosphere and environment as possible, within which the necessary level of nursing care can be safely and efficiently provided. Even the most frail or heavily dependent residents should be able to maintain their dignity. The current trend is to provide individual personal space for residents. Hence, individual rooms with toilet facilities en-suite backed-up by communal lounges and dining areas along with shared treatment and assisted bathing rooms are the norm. Special attention is required to making sure the facilities are suitable for the physically disabled and frail.

Typically, the following facilities are required:

- A reassuring and welcoming entrance and reception facility for arriving visitors and potential new residents.
- An office for the 'head of home' and a general administration office, both close to the main entrance.
- A staff base or bases in central positions relative to bedroom clusters. This is particularly important at night.
- Bedrooms, each of which should be for a single resident except for one or two double rooms for married couples. Rooms should be capable of accommodating some personal possessions and furniture. Space must be provided for wheelchair maneuvering, the use of walking aids and hoists, and assistance by staff. A choice of positions for beds and furniture is desirable. Provision for clothes, both handing and in drawers,

must be made. Space is required for one or two easy chairs, a moveable table and a dressing table that can be used as a writing desk. Each bedroom should have direct access to a room with a WC, washbasin and a bath or shower.

In addition other rooms are required within easy reach of bedrooms. They include the following:

- An assisted bathing room (with access to three sides of the bath) and assisted showering. These rooms should have hair-washing facilities and be capable of accommodating wheelchairs. The number of residents and the location of the rooms in relation to the bedrooms they serve, especially if the bedrooms are on more than one floor, should determine the number of these rooms.
- A secure treatment/clinical room with associated secure storage for clean linen, drugs, medicines, sterile and disposable supplies.
- A room for emptying, cleaning and disinfecting bedpans, for urine testing samples, for temporary holding of items for disposal or reprocessing, and for the parking of wheelchairs and/or commodes.
- Rooms for communal dining and sitting, and alcoves or similar for more private conversation.
- Beverage preparation bays convenient to the bedrooms so that residents can entertain visitors in their rooms.
- A kitchen located and designed to easily receive deliveries and for rapid serving and distribution of food to the dining areas and bedrooms.
- A laundry, including provision for receiving and sorting heavily soiled linen, for washing, spin and tumble drying, pressing folding and sorting, marking and repairing.

- One central domestic services base and outstations as necessary on each floor to accommodate cleaning equipment, trolleys and materials.
- A disposal room near a service entrance for sealed containers for refuse and reprocessing items.
- A small room to serve as a mortuary, convenient for discreet access by hearse.
- Staff facilities, including separate toilets for male and female staff, dining and rest areas, changing rooms, lockers and staff showers.
- General storage and maintenance provisions.

LARGE HOSPITALS

OPD

Location

- It is situated for convenience and accessibility of inpatients and outpatients.
- Wall mounted signboards must be used for the assistance of new patients.
- Pediatric clinic is close to the entrance to reduce travel distance for the mother carrying an infant.
- New patients should be directed to the admitting interview cubicle.
- Appropriate waiting place must be provided for patients waiting prescription from the pharmacy dispensary.
- Appropriate spaces and fixtures should be provided for handicapped persons.
- Each examination room has minimum 80 net sq.ft. usable floor area.
- Treatment rooms shall have minimum 120 net sq.ft. usable floor space.

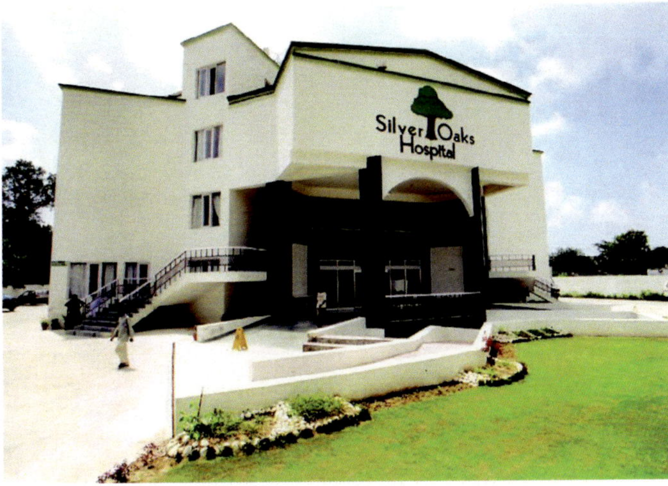

Fig. 5.8: Silver Oaks Hospital at Mohali, Punjab

- Examination tables must be accessible on 3 sides allowing for working space on each side.
- Each room should have a lavatory, sufficient room for the patients changing area, examination table, doctor's desk, an X-ray viewing box.
- There should be phone outlet and remote dictation electronic intercom-between each room and outpatient control station.

Out-Patient's Department (OPD) and Services

The OPD provides consultation, investigation and diagnoses for patients who required little or no recovery services afterwards and generally attended by appointment. There is usually a main waiting area, with registration and enquiry point, but, preferably, it should be relatively small, with patients sent onwards to sub-waiting

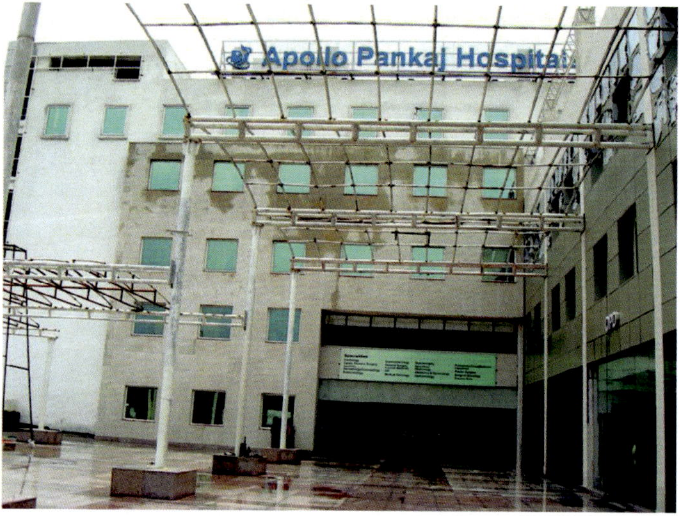

Fig. 5.9: Apollo Pankaj Hospital, Agra

areas near the clinic they are to attend. Those clinics with little specialized equipment (e.g. general medicines, general surgery, gynecology, urology) can use multipurpose consulting and examining facilities. Although traditionally many doctors preferred a purpose-designed clinic, with designated consulting rooms, each with one or more examining rooms, a more flexible and economical arrangement is a long row or string of combined consulting and examining (CE) rooms, in which the patient remains in one room, but the doctor may move between two or three adjoining rooms. Each should be 14 to 15 m^2, with sound resisting intercommunicating doors. Each clinic will use as many CE rooms as its staff and patients need.

The key to economy in construction and efficiency in use is to plan for 85 or 90 percent occupancy. This is easier to achieve in multipurpose OP suites than for clinics like ophthalmology, which require much specialized equipment, and which are not easy (and not usually appropriate) to use for other purposes. Associated with each group of CE rooms should be a sub-waiting space, nurse's treatment room, with clean and dirty utility rooms, toilets and weighing and measuring facilities. A toilet adjoining a dirty utility room can have a pass-through hatch for specimen testing.

Some clinics can use CE rooms for most purposes, but also need some special accommodation to serve cardiac clinics (e.g. electrocardiography (ECG)), audiology (a soundproof room-often a prefabricated booth) for ear and throat clinics, and treatment baths and ultra-violet light equipment for dermatology. Genito-urinary clinics deal with veneral diseases and used to be discreetly located away from all other hospital functions, although this is not now generally deemed necessary, and they may be part of a general OPD. They are often open at evenings and weekends, and so access must take this into account. They also keep extensive records and they can share facilities with the dermatology clinics, and may be adjacent to them. Fracture and orthopedic clinics are often planned in association with the A & E department, for sharing of plaster room and of staff. Both in waiting area, toilets, CE and other clinical rooms, the space required by people with disabilities and those with limbs in plaster will be greater than in most other areas.

Children may attend any of the clinics at an OPD, but as far as possible they should have separate provision. This may be combined with a child assessment center for investigating possible anomalies of development; this requires facilities for testing sight, hearing, speech, mobility and intelligence. Antenatal clinics may be associated with (but distinct from) those for gynecology, or form part of a maternity department. In some hospital with a patient-focused emphasis, both may form part of a 'women's and children's unit'.

Accident and Emergency (A & E)

Various studies have indicated that only around 1 percent of those attending an accident and emergency department are suffering from major trauma needing a high level of multi-disciplinary care and, at the other end of the scale, around 50 percent of attendees could more appropriately have been treated by their GP. This has led to a move to provide a wider range of A & E facilities from regional major trauma centers, through departments in local hospitals down to enhanced facilities in local GP-based centers. Because the term 'trauma center' has a number of different interpretations, the term A & E is used here to describe all types of facility. Much of the accommodation required for a 'minor accident unit' (MAU) in a local hospital is of a similar nature, but is smaller, simpler and with less specialized equipment.

For all types of A & E or MAU the entrance provides the first impression of the hospital for the most ill and anxious patients, and their equally anxious family and friends. While they may not be consciously aware of the appearance of the building it is likely to be one factor that will increase or lessen their anxiety. Also very important is the signposting both to the hospital and within the hospital's grounds. In most cases, and certainly for trauma centers, a helicopter-landing pad will be needed, as close as possible to the A & E's entrance.

Traditionally, two entrances are provided, one for the 'walking wounded' and one for ambulance cases. For an MAU, only one is needed; the same may be argued for a trauma center-type A & E. In all cases, a substantial draught lobby is required with automatic doors at each end. These should preferably be at right angles to each other, to prevent both opening together and thus causing a through draught; this requires generous space for turning. In areas where violence or disturbances are common the inner doors from the draught lobby may be locked from the reception point, to keep out those who may be trying to continue an affray. A single entrance reduces ambiguity or confusion as to where people should go. If the draught lobby is overlooked from the reception point, those entering may be directed either to the waiting area, or immediately to the resuscitation and treatment areas.

The sorting of patients according to the urgency of their need is referred to as 'triage'. Initial triage is usually undertaken by an experienced nurse, whose base should enable him/her to observe everyone while entering and to make a preliminary assessment of their condition. A small room adjoining both, the base and the reception counter, will facilitate confidential interviews.

Registration usually takes place after the triage nurse has seen the patient; in the case of seriously ill or injured patients, it will take place later.

In cases where there is a single entrance, once inside the A & E's draught lobby the two streams of patients should be separated. The serious emergency case will go straight to the resuscitation room (with medical gases and X-ray facilities) or major treatment room (sometimes referred to as a minor theater). In the case of the A & E of a traditional DGH, the number of places in the resuscitation room will depend on the population served, and this is reflected in the annual attendances; a range of 3000 to 70,000 is typical, although a number of large urban hospitals now have attendance of more than 100,000. In the instance of trauma centers backed up by MAUs, the resuscitation room will be sized according to the number of serious emergency cases.

Patients with less urgent conditions will go after triage and registration to a waiting area that must be as quiet, comfortably furnished and attractive as possible. Children and their parents should be directed immediately to a separate waiting area with associated examination, treatment and consulting rooms. All other patients will be called forward to one of a range of cubicles or rooms. Most will need to be examined and treated on a couch. For some, a smaller cubicle for seated treatment is adequate. Separate rooms will be needed for eye injuries, for distressed or noisy patients, or those with alcohol or drug problems. A room for the application of plasters may be shared with the fracture and orthopedic clinic. Emergency X-ray facilities may form part of the A & E, but are more economic if they can form part of a nearby imaging department.

The size of the main waiting room will depend on the extent to which patients are called forward to sub-waiting areas. It needs public telephones, and some facilities for refreshments, unless it is close to the cafes at the main entrance. Such proximity make for ease of operation at night, as the A & E entrance may well then be the only one open. Outside the building, there must be sufficient separation of traffic routes, so that the A & E access route is not blocked-a few parking spaces are needed nearby for cars bringing emergency patients, but parking and unloading space for ambulances takes priority.

Intensive Therapy, Coronary Care and High-Dependency Units

The term Intensive Therapy Unit (rather than intensive care unit) denotes active medical as well as nursing treatment of those most at risk, either following surgery, accidents or sudden illness such as strokes. The unit should be in close proximity to operating theaters and easily accessible from the accident and emergency department and in-patient areas generally. A large space is required for each bed, together with extensive services that need to be located in such a way as to allow free movement of staff around the bed and to the patient. Various methods have been used for providing these services and experience suggests that they are best delivered from overhead by swiveled pendant or service beam, which leave the floor around the bed free for staff and resuscitation and other equipment. Patients are continuously monitored and the monitoring apparatus must be in clear view. Supplies may be held on mobile shelf units of sufficient height between adjacent beds while also allowing standing staff to have a generally clear view around the multi-bed area. A few beds should be in single rooms to cater for cases needing isolation because of infection or other reasons.

A Coronary Care Unit (CCU) can be similarly equipped for patients who have suffered coronaries. In very large hospitals, the CCU may be associated with the cardiac medical and surgical departments. In other hospitals, the ITU and CCU may be a twinned unit sharing facilities such as supplies, on-call accommodation for staff and waiting areas for relatives. More single rooms are required for CCU beds in order to provide a minimum stress environment.

A High-Dependency Unit (HDU) may be a part of a group of ordinary wards with higher staffing for the most ill patients, or may be associated with the ITU, providing a 'step-down' from that unit. However, with shorter stay, most hospital in patients can be regarded as high-dependency, and thus distinction is becoming less valid.

ITUs and CCUs are accepted as suitable for male and female patients being located in the same bed area. However, in hospitals with a large children's unit, a separate children's ITU is desirable and justified.

There is evidence that patients who appear to be semi-conscious may be aware of their surroundings and remember their experiences to a surprising degree. In spite of the inevitable omnipresence of high-technology equipment, much care must be given to making the environment as pleasant as possible. Good external views are important in order to help ease patient anxiety and relieve the stressful nature of the work for the staff.

Chapter 6

Alternative Healing Methods

HOLISTIC AND ALTERNATIVE MEDICINES

Apart from relying on modern technology and medicines, holistic medicine welcomes all the techniques that have been developed in other cultures and at other times. Holistic is derived from the ancient Greek word "holos" which means whole. It was first introduced by the South African statesman and biologist Jan Christian Smuts in his book Holism and Evolution as early as in 1926. Holistic medicine is also an alternative to scientific approach that attempts to understand all phenomena including human beings. Thus, it makes use of a variety of therapeutic approaches. These have been described as "alternative" or complementary medicine, e.g. reiki, crystal healing, sujok, acupuncture, acupressure, panchkarma oil massage, yoga, Indian mudras, homopathy, ayurveda, naturopathy and many more. Twist and smile meditation recently introduced by Prof. Parkjae Woo who has enriched our knowledge by the therapeutic correspondence systems of the hands and feet also has abundance cure effect of our ailments. These are most popular methods that being highly effective, easy to learn and use, safe, cost-efficient and time sparing. These are drugless, non-medication methods and treatment.

AYURVEDA

Spatial Requirements

Dhara

Dhara is good for all diseases. There are varieties of Dhara. They are mainly grouped as Moordhanya (on the head), Sarvangeena (all over the body) and Pradeshika (local). The most important and commonly done is Moordhanya.

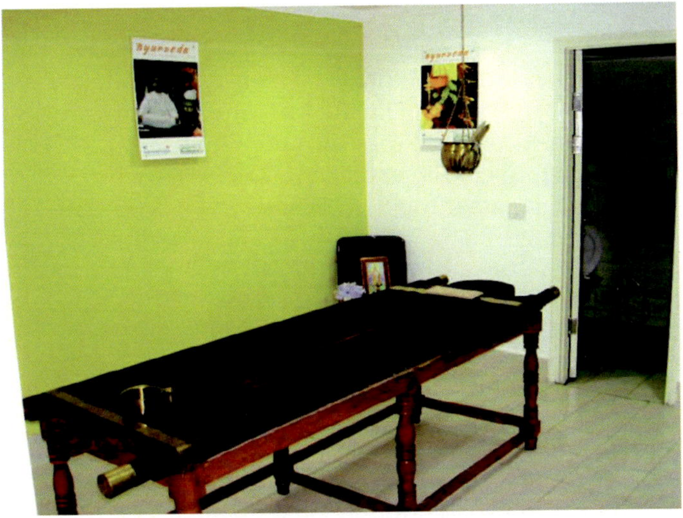

Fig. 6.1: The traditional Kerala massage table

This is usually performed by 2-3 attendants and a physician. Dhara is generally done for 7 to 14 days. Shirodhara is usually never done for more than 21 days.

A Dharapathi/droni

The first requirement is the proper droni. Many trees such as Deodar, Pine, Punnaga, Mango tree are recommended for this. The ideal wood universally accepted by physicians is Nuxvomica. Jack and Asana (Madras Kino) are also good. Average dharapathi must be 55-80 cm in breath and 2.5 to 3 m in length. There is a pit to which liquid flows when dhara is conducted. There is a hole to the pit which allow liquid to flow out. There should be handles on all the four corners 12 to 24 cm long to help to carry droni. The height of supports is 24 to 36 cm. The droni is usually oriented in east-west direction.

Dharachatti

These vessels are used for Dhara, is usually made of clay. The edge of vessel is to be thick and turned outwards, so that it is easy to tie the rope around it for hanging. A hole is bored in the very center of the vessel and a wick of thread is allowed to pass through it. The liquid is allowed to flow down through this hole.

Other Requirements

- Space for burner for heating oil
- Storage of towels, oil, etc.
- Fixture for the dharachatti
- Changing room/toilet facility
- Three small seats for physician and attendants
- Circulation space around Dharapathi
- A vessel to collect dhara liquid coming out of droni
- Two suitable receptacles to receive liquid and pour it again into Dhara vessel
- A time keeper (clock).

Njavarakizhi (Pindaswedam)

Pindasweda is a rejuvenation technique that causes the entire body to perspire by using medicinal puddings. Four practitioners are required along with a supervisor and an attendant who heats and replaces the boluses. Out of the eight bundles, four of them are removed from simmering liquid and left to cool for five minutes. While the four bundles are used, the remaining four are kept heated in the decoction. As the bundles cool, the attendant replaces them with the warm ones and re-heats the cool boluses. The attendant ensures that no interruption occurs during abhyanga. This is generally done for 7, 9, 11 or 14 days.

Requirements

- A droni
- Seating space for 4 attendants, physician
- Space for burner
- Storage space for towels, pans
- Changing room/toilet
- Circulation space around droni

Pizhichil

This form of abhyanga is said to be most beneficial for rejuvenating the nervous system. In this method, the medicated oil used is poured over the person's body from a height of 15 angula (head) and 13 angula (body), while simultaneously being rubbed into the body. Four practitioners attend the seated person. Two practitioners massage from shoulders to navel, and the other two practitioners massage from navel to the feet. In this approach, clothes are soaked in oil/ghee and squeezed on the body. A fifth practitioner keeps the clothes in warm oil and replaces them as they cool off. Generally the person receives the massage for one hour. If the treatment lasts for 14 or 21 days, the time of each session is gradually increased.

Requirements

- A droni
- Space for burner to heat oil
- Storage space for towels, pans
- Changing room/toilet
- Circulation space around droni
- Enough space for attendants

Psychiatric

- A discrete but linked block to District General Hospital.
- Linked with local population so that community health worked interact with mental health team psychiatrists, psychiatric nurses, occupational therapist, social workers.
- Most people presenting symptoms of mental illness are treated as out-patients/day patients.
- Size depends on DGH-60 to 150 beds.
- Facility for individual, group, occupational therapy.
- Units favor single bedroom-small-but not for dangerous illness.
- Elderly-diagnosis of psychological systems, generally deteriorative diseases is done on out-patient basis.
- Patients of depression are cared for in general psychial units.

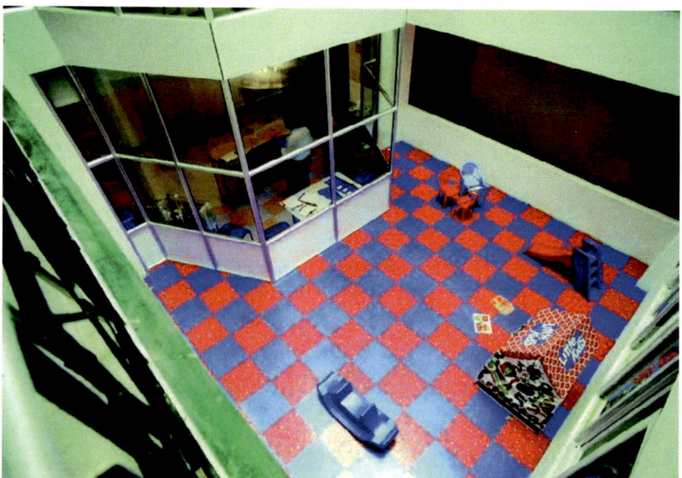

Fig. 6.2: An interesting play area for children for recuperating

- With advanced dementia—need protected nursing home environment are ambulant—secure in outdoor walking space.
- Day area need wide range of rooms-planned 2B highly adaptable comfy sitting-1 to 1 therapy, interview, group therapy training-100 ms has observation three 1 way window.
- Heavy workshops, craft, psycotherapy, outdoor needed in longer stay units.

What is Reiki?

Reiki is universal life force energy. Reiki is God's love in purest form.

Reiki is a thousand year old healing technique. It is a natural healing system based on ancient Tibetian Buddhist Scriptures. It heals of mental, emotional problems as well as minor acute and chronic physical problems. It promotes relaxation, vitality and positivity. It helps us to face the changes of life and keep away stress, anxiety and depression.

Reiki is the radiant healing touch for health, happiness and prosperity.

Brief History of Reiki

Dr Mikao Usui was the founder of the modern day Reiki. Towards the end of 19th century, Dr Usui lived in Kyoto, Japan. He was a Christian Minister and the Principal of Doshisha University. When some students asked him to demonstrate how Jesus Christ healed people, he was inspired to investigate the phenomenon of healing because he was ignorant of that. He left the job, travelled to Chicago, USA where he received a doctorate in Theology. He went to China, Tibet and learnt Chinese so as to study translation, still without success. Back to Japan, he visited Buddhist monasteries to learn scriptures. He learned Sanskrit, the original language to pursue the Buddhist sutras that had never been translated. Finally Dr Usui found the formula, the symbols, and the key to healing in Lotus sutra.

In 1914 after meditating on the sacred mountain of Koriyama for 21 days, the meaning and the use of these symbols were revealed to him. Thus, the USUI system of Reiki was rediscovered.

Reiki is not a religion. It has no dogma. It has nothing to do with spiritualism, occultism, demons, ghosts, hypnosis, etc. people of all age can learn Reiki.

Some results of Reiki treatments

- It heals holistically
- Relieves, stress, strain and tension
- Helps relieve insomnia
- Harmonises body and mind
- Enhances intuitive powers
- Develops self confidence.

What can be Treated?

It actually works to enhance the effectiveness of all other types of therapy. Reiki can be the first step towards realizing self. It is a beautiful experience and helps in Sadhna. Spiritual growth is not possible if you are sick-physically or mentally. In its long history of use it has aided in healing virtuality every known disease and injuries including serious problems like multiple sclerosis, heart diseases, cancer, skin problems, cuts, bruises, headache, sore throat, fatigue, poor memory, lack of confidence, cold, flu and impotency. If a client has a health condition and wants to treat with Reiki, it is recommended to consult the doctor. Reiki will improve the results of all medical treatment, shortens healing time and eliminates pain.

Attunement Process

Reiki is transferred to the student by the Reiki master through the attunement process—a secret and sacred technique. It is a powerful and spiritual experience. It creates a special link between the student and the Reiki source. It is also attended by Reiki guides who help in implementing the process. Many feel mystical experience, healing, vision and past life experiences—opening of the third eye, intuitive awareness. Energy flow coming from the cosmos down to the Crown Chakra, Third Eye Chakra, Throat Chakra, Heart Chakra and flow to its natural extension, the hands.

DEGREES

There are four degrees of Reiki.

First Degree

Attunement focuses on elevating the energy of the physical body. It enables a person to notice and feel the sensation of energy in his hands. It treats and heals the ailments, calms the mind and relaxes the nerves. It open four chakras.

Second Degree

Reiki gives attunement for higher level of energy. It works on etheric body. It imparts symbols which are used to perform absentee, mental and emotional healing. It intensifies the effect of Reiki treatment. Second degree Reiki can go beyond time and space. It releases the negative conditioning from the past experiences, cleans the environment, smoothes out journey/travels. It harmonises relationship. It enables us to remove mental blocks. It is to liberate the mind stream from the shackles of long buried memories and emotions. When exposed to the power of universal life force energy, those remnants of old traumas and misunderstanding can no longer cling to us. In addition, three sacred symbols which act as focus points for the mind to enable the practitioner to create a bridge from his heart to the heart of other, over which the energy can be drawn, we are enabled to give distant treatments across space and also forward or backward in time.

Third Degree
Reiki attunement is given with the most powerful symbol, above all the other symbols.

Fourth Degree
It is teacher's attunement. If you are really dedicated and committed to teach and have done lots of healing, you may go in for fourth degree. You have to empty the empty cup. Your ego steps out of the way. When you are a true Reiki master you understand that everything is equal by the life force energy. In this spirit of absolute equality, you became a mirror to your students, mirroring back to them the truth of who they are. "It is a high level, deep meditation wherein we invoke cosmic energy in our body through the chakras to energise our physical, mental, emotional, intellectual and spiritual bodies".

FIVE PRINCIPLES OF REIKI

- Just for today, I will not fear.
- Just for today, I will not anger.
- Just for today, I will honour my parents, teachers and elders.
- Just for today, I will earn my living honestly.
- Just for today, I shall show gratitude towards everything.

How it Works?

Reiki open the blockages and circulates the free flow of energy. This energy nourishes our organs and glands and we regain health, happiness and relaxation. Reiki heals by calming the mind and raising the life force energy in the body.

The Seven Chakras

To understand Reiki better an understanding of the Chakras or the major energy centers located around the spine is important. Chakra is Sanskrit word, means wheel or disk. The energy centers nourish our organs and glands. There are seven key chakras in the human body–Muldhara, Swadhishthana, Manipura, Anahata, Vishuddha, Ajna and Pituitary.

The chakras may get blocked due to emotional, physical or spiritual problems. Reiki works on energy centers, and remove the blockages and creates balance. Thus, it is a effective healing method in all kinds of illness in conjunction with all other medical and therapeutic techniques.

- Reiki touch – touches the HEART
- Reiki touch – Soothes the MIND
- Reiki touch – Heals the BODY
- Reiki touches the FEELINGS which need to be felt
- Reiki touch empowers yourself to HIGHERSELF (Geeta Sharma and Shivani Sharma).

To sum up Reiki empowers each man to make his life fruitful, living in harmony with the biorhythms of nature, channelizing his own unique, unlimited internal resources to attain complete health and unfurl his full potential.

Index

G

H

I

L

M

N

O

P

R

S

V

W